Raising Your ADHD Teenage Boy: Transforming Chaos to Calm, Parenting Your Son

I Booky

All rights reserved. No part of this publication may be reproduced, distributed, or transmitted in any form or by any means, including photocopying, recording, or other electronic or mechanical methods, without the prior written permission of the publisher, except in the case of brief quotations embodied in critical reviews and certain other noncommercial uses permitted by copyright law.

Copyright © I Booky, 2023.

Disclaimer

The content of this book, "Raising Your ADHD Teenage Boy: Transforming Chaos to Calm, Parenting Your Son," is provided for educational purposes only. While every effort has been made to ensure accuracy, the author and publisher do not guarantee the completeness, accuracy, or suitability of the information.

The author and publisher disclaim any liability for the use or application of the information contained in this book. Readers are encouraged to use their discretion and judgment when applying the content. By reading this book, you agree to these terms and conditions.

Transforming Chaos to Calm, Parenting Your Son / I Booky

Free Bonus

Successful Keys to Help your Son Stay Calm and Make Smarter Choices

1. Encourage regular physical activity to release excess energy.
2. Practice deep breathing exercises to promote relaxation.
3. Establish consistent daily routines and schedules.
4. Use visual aids and reminders for tasks and deadlines.
5. Provide a quiet and organized study environment.
6. Break tasks into smaller, manageable steps.
7. Set clear and achievable goals.
8. Teach problem-solving skills to address challenges.
9. Encourage positive self-talk and affirmations.

10. Foster open communication and active listening.
11. Promote healthy sleep habits and routines.
12. Implement mindfulness and meditation practices.
13. Teach time management and prioritization skills.
14. Limit screen time and electronic device use.
15. Encourage journaling or creative expression for emotional release.
16. Provide healthy snacks and meals to support brain function.
17. Model calm and positive behavior in stressful situations.
18. Use positive reinforcement and praise for good behavior.
19. Offer choices to empower decision-making.
20. Provide opportunities for physical outlets, such as sports or hobbies.
21. Teach relaxation techniques, such as progressive muscle relaxation.

22. Implement a reward system for achieving goals.
23. Encourage social connections and friendships.
24. Teach problem-solving and conflict resolution skills.
25. Foster a sense of independence and autonomy.
26. Create a safe and supportive home environment.
27. Seek professional guidance and support from therapists or counselors.
28. Practice patience and understanding during challenging moments.
29. Encourage participation in extracurricular activities or clubs.
30. Establish clear rules and boundaries with consistent consequences.
31. Teach self-regulation techniques, such as counting to ten before reacting.
32. Provide opportunities for creative expression, such as art or music.
33. Offer choices for relaxation activities, such as reading or listening to music.

34. Model healthy coping strategies for stress and anxiety.
35. Teach problem-solving skills for managing conflicts with peers.
36. Encourage regular breaks during homework or study sessions.
37. Foster a sense of belonging and acceptance at home and school.
38. Provide opportunities for hands-on learning and exploration.
39. Offer praise and recognition for effort, not just outcomes.
40. Teach assertiveness skills for advocating for oneself.
41. Encourage positive relationships with teachers and peers.
42. Practice active listening and empathy during conversations.
43. Foster resilience and perseverance in the face of setbacks.
44. Teach organization skills for managing belongings and schoolwork.
45. Provide opportunities for reflection and self-assessment.

46. Offer support and encouragement during transitions or changes.
47. Model healthy coping strategies for managing emotions.
48. Encourage involvement in community service or volunteer work.
49. Provide opportunities for leadership and responsibility.
50. Celebrate successes and milestones along the way.

By implementing these successful keys, you can help your ADHD teen son stay calm, focused, and make smarter choices in various aspects of his life.

Table of Contents

Free Bonus — 5
   Successful Keys to Help your Son Stay Calm and Make Smarter Choices — 5
INTRODUCTION — 15
   ● Why this Book is Necessary — 16
   ● What to Expect from this Book — 18
   ● Understanding ADHD in Teen Boys — 19
      ➔ THE INATTENTIVE TYPE OF ADHD IN TEEN BOYS — 23
      ➔ Hyperactive-impulsive type of ADHD in teen boys — 24
      ➔ Combined type — 26
   ● DIAGNOSIS — 28
   ● Principles of Parenting a Teen Boy with ADHD — 31
   ● Assessment Questions to Determine if Your Teen Boy Has ADHD — 33
   ● Things Your Teen Boy Wishes You Knew About ADHD — 36
Chapter 1 — 41
   TAKING CHARGE OF ADHD IN YOUR TEEN BOY — 41
      ● How to Take Charge of ADHD in Your Teen Boy — 42
      ● Safe Care Tips for Your Teen Boy with ADHD — 57
      ● Prioritizing Yourself as a Parent of a Teen Boy with ADHD — 59
      ● Responding Appropriately to Different

    Behavioral Situations   61
- Identifying Your Teen Boy's Triggers   63
- Handling Explosive Behavior Without Losing Control   65
- Developing Social Awareness and Responsibility in Your Teen Boy   67

Chapter 2   71
HYPERACTIVITY   71
- What Causes Hyperactivity in Teen Boys with Adhd?   71
- How does hyperactivity affect daily life?   72
- Physical symptoms: 74
- Behavioral symptoms: 74
- Emotional symptoms: 75
- The diagnosis process   75
- Treatment options   77
- Alternative treatments and therapies   79
- Lifestyle Changes to Manage Hyperactivity   80
  → Diet and nutrition tips   80
  → Exercise and physical activity recommendations   82
  → Sleep and relaxation strategies   83

Chapter 3   85
IMPULSIVITY   85
- Impulsivity as a symptom of ADHD   85
- Importance of understanding impulsivity in teen boys with ADHD   86
- Impact of impulsivity on daily life   88
- Impact of impulsivity on daily life   90

- Causes of Impulsivity in Teen Boys with ADHD 90
  - Environmental factors 91
  - Neurological factors 93
- Managing Impulsivity in Teen Boys with ADHD 93
  - Medication 93
  - Behavioral therapy 94
  - Cognitive-behavioral therapy 95
  - Parent training 95
- School-based interventions 95
- Strategies for Coping with Impulsivity 96
  - Mindfulness techniques 97
  - Relaxation techniques 97
  - Organization and planning strategies 97
  - Exercise and physical activity 97
  - Support groups 98

Chapter 4 99
INATTENTION 99
- Definition 99
- Importance of Addressing Inattention in Teen Boys with ADHD 99
- Signs and Symptoms 101
- Differences between Inattention in ADHD and Typical Teenage Behaviors 102
- Factors Contributing to Inattention in Teen Boys with ADHD 103
- Behavioral Interventions 106
- Medication Management 108

- → Types of Medications for ADHD — 108
- → Side Effects and Risks — 109
- Medication Compliance — 110
- Psychotherapy — 110
- Educational Support — 113
- Tips for Parenting a Teen Boy with Inattention in ADHD — 114

Conclusion — 116

Chapter 5 — 119
STRATEGIES FOR DAILY LIFE — 119
- Creating Routines and Schedules that Work — 119
- Managing Time and Priorities — 120
- Helping Your Teen Boy Stay Organized — 122
- Promoting Healthy Habits for Success — 123
- Improving Sleep Habits — 125
- Navigating Social Situations and Friendships — 127
- Helping Your Teen Boy Manage Screen Time — 129

Chapter 6 — 131
ACADEMIC SUCCESS — 131
- Supporting Learning at Home — 131
- Strategies for Success at School — 133
- Managing Home Assignments — 141
- Preparing for Tests and Exams — 143
- Navigating the IEP and 504 Process — 145
- Working with Teachers and Other Professionals — 147

Chapter 7   151
    EMOTIONAL WELL-BEING   151
- Understanding Emotional Regulation in Teen Boys with ADHD   151
- Strategies for Managing Emotional Outbursts   154
- Helping Your Teen Boy Build Self-Esteem and Confidence   156
- Coping with Anxiety and Depression   158
- Supporting Positive Relationships with Family and Peers   160
- Navigating the Challenges of Puberty   162

Chapter 8   165
    PLANNING FOR THE FUTURE   165
- Preparing for Life After High School   165
- Post-Secondary Education and Training Options   167
- Preparing for the Workforce   170
- Building Life Skills for Independence   171
- Navigating the Transition to Adulthood   174

CONCLUSION   177
Other Books by the Same Author   179

INTRODUCTION

Do you feel like you're constantly struggling to make things work for your teenage son with ADHD? Do you ever ask why he can't listen or behave like other teens his age? It can be frustrating, and sometimes it may feel like there is no end in sight.

But what if I told you that there's hope? You can find the strength and guidance to help your son survive and thrive in this challenging world.

Welcome to this book on raising a teenage boy with ADHD. It's not just another parenting guide but a beacon of hope for you if you feel you are at the end of your rope. In this book, you'll discover insights, tips, and strategies curated carefully and intentionally.

You'll learn to navigate the tough times with compassion and grace, build stronger connections with your son, and create a home environment that fosters growth and learning.

But more than that, this book speaks to the heart of parenting. It acknowledges the doubts, fears, and struggles you face as a parent and encourages you to embrace your imperfections and cultivate deep compassion for yourself and your son.

You're not alone on this journey and don't have to do it alone. This book will be a source of inspiration and support, a reminder that you can be great with the proper guidance. So let's dive in together and discover what's possible when approaching parenting with intention, curiosity, and love.

- **Why this Book is Necessary**

Parenting is an arduous journey, full of highs and lows, twists and turns. As parents, we all want the best for our children, but the path to success sometimes seems unclear and overwhelming. In today's world, where children face increasing demands and pressures, it's more important than ever to equip ourselves with the skills and knowledge to help them navigate the challenges they will face.

That's where this book comes in. It's a guidebook for parents who want to raise emotionally intelligent children - children who can communicate effectively, build strong relationships, and navigate the complexities of modern life with confidence and grace. Through this book, you will gain a deeper understanding of the importance of emotional intelligence and discover practical strategies for fostering emotional growth and well-being in your child.

This book is necessary because it offers a roadmap for you to give your son the best possible start in life. It's a guide that will help you navigate the ups and downs of parenting and equip you with the tools you need to raise happy, successful, and emotionally intelligent sons. This book is a must-read to help your child thrive in today's fast-paced and complex world.

So let's embark on this journey together and discover the transformative power of emotional intelligence.

• What to Expect from this Book

This book is a comprehensive guide that provides you with practical advice, strategies, and tools to raise emotionally intelligent children. In the following pages, you will find valuable insights on creating a safe and nurturing environment for your child to grow and develop.

Through engaging and interactive exercises, you will learn how to identify and manage your emotions effectively, which will help you model healthy emotional regulation for your son. You will also discover how to communicate effectively with your son, build strong relationships, and foster empathy and social skills.

Furthermore, you will also understand how to support your child's unique personality and strengths while helping him overcome any limitations or challenges he may face.

But this book isn't just about solving problems – it's about unlocking the full potential of your child. You'll learn how to support your son's unique personality and strengths, while also helping him overcome any limitations or challenges he may face. And as he grows and develops, you'll discover how to help him stay organized and independent, preparing him for a successful and fulfilling future.

Overall, this book is a valuable resource for you if you want to raise an emotionally intelligent son and provides a roadmap for building strong, healthy, and fulfilling relationships with your teenage son.

- **Understanding ADHD in Teen Boys**

Attention-deficit/hyperactivity disorder (ADHD) is a common neurodevelopmental disorder affecting children and adults. Now we will focus on understanding ADHD in teen boys, including the causes, symptoms, and treatment options.

Firstly, it's essential to understand that ADHD is not caused by poor parenting or bad behavior. ADHD is a complex condition that arises from genetic, environmental, and neurological factors.

Research has shown that genetics play a significant role in the development of ADHD. Studies have found that if a parent or sibling has ADHD, the chances of another family member developing the disorder are much higher than in families without a history of ADHD.

It has also been found that certain genes are associated with ADHD. For example, genes involved in the regulation of dopamine, a neurotransmitter in the brain that affects motivation and reward, have been linked to ADHD. In addition, genes related to the development and function of the prefrontal cortex, a part of the brain involved in executive functions such as attention, working memory, and impulse control, have also been identified as potential contributors to ADHD.

It's important to note, however, that genetics are not the sole cause of ADHD.

While genetics cannot be changed, understanding the role they play in ADHD can help parents and individuals with ADHD better manage their symptoms and seek appropriate treatment. It can also help to reduce stigma and promote understanding of the disorder as a neurological condition rather than a result of poor parenting or personal weakness.

However, certain environmental factors such as prenatal exposure to alcohol, premature birth, and low birth weight may increase the risk of developing ADHD. Additionally, certain lifestyle factors such as poor nutrition, lack of physical activity, and exposure to high levels of stress can exacerbate symptoms of ADHD.

ADHD symptoms can vary from person to person. They can be classified into three types: inattentive, hyperactive-impulsive, and combined. Teen boys with ADHD typically exhibit hyperactive-impulsive symptoms, such as restlessness, fidgeting, interrupting, and impulsivity. They may also need help with inattention, such as forgetfulness, disorganization, and distractibility.

It's essential to note that ADHD can significantly impact a teen's academic performance, social relationships, and emotional well-being. Teen boys with ADHD are at higher risk of developing depression, anxiety, and other mental health problems.

The good news is that ADHD is treatable, and early intervention can significantly improve outcomes. Treatment options may include medication, behavioral therapy, or a combination of both.

Understanding ADHD in teen boys is crucial to ensure early diagnosis, intervention, and treatment. By identifying and addressing ADHD symptoms, you can help your son with ADHD achieve his full potential and improve his quality of life.

→ THE INATTENTIVE TYPE OF ADHD IN TEEN BOYS

The inattentive type of ADHD in teen boys is characterized by symptoms such as difficulty sustaining attention, being forgetful, being disorganized, and being easily distracted. Teen boys with inattentive ADHD may struggle to follow instructions, finish tasks, or pay attention to details. They may also need help to stay on task or complete homework assignments on time.

In addition to academic difficulties, the inattentive type of ADHD can also impact your son's social life. He will struggle to maintain friendships or have difficulty participating in group activities due to his inability to focus or stay on task.

You must recognize the signs and symptoms of inattentive ADHD in your son to provide appropriate support and intervention. With the correct diagnosis and treatment, your son with inattentive ADHD will learn strategies to manage his symptoms and thrive academically, socially, and emotionally.

➔ **Hyperactive-impulsive type of ADHD in teen boys**

Hyperactive-impulsive type of ADHD in teen boys is another subtype of ADHD that is characterized by hyperactivity and impulsivity. Boys with this subtype are often very fidgety and restless and have difficulty sitting still for extended periods. They may also be very talkative, interrupt others, and have difficulty waiting their turn.

Teen boys with hyperactive-impulsive type ADHD often act before thinking, which can lead to impulsive behavior such as blurting out answers in class or making impulsive decisions. They may also have difficulty regulating emotions, leading to outbursts of temper tantrums.

This subtype of ADHD can also present challenges in social situations, as hyperactive-impulsive symptoms can make it difficult to form and maintain friendships. Teachers and parents may also have difficulty managing the behaviors of a teen boy with hyperactive-impulsive type ADHD, as they may be disruptive in the classroom or at home.

You must understand the unique challenges associated with hyperactive-impulsive type ADHD in teen boys to provide appropriate support and interventions. A combination of medication and therapy effectively manages and improves symptoms.

➔ Combined type

A combined type of ADHD is a condition that affects many teen boys. Both inattentive and hyperactive-impulsive symptoms characterize this type of ADHD. Teen boys with combined type ADHD may struggle with staying focused and paying attention to tasks, as well as with impulsive behavior and difficulty sitting still.

Some common symptoms of combined-type ADHD in teen boys include trouble following through with tasks, forgetfulness, disorganization, interrupting others, fidgeting or squirming, and difficulty staying seated. Teen boys with this type of ADHD may struggle to regulate their emotions and have frequent outbursts or mood swings.

With the right interventions, your son with the combined type ADHD will learn to manage his symptoms and thrive in school, relationships, and other areas of life.

Symptoms

ADHD symptoms can significantly affect a teenager's life and make completing tasks and following through with responsibilities challenging. The symptoms of ADHD can be grouped into two categories: inattention and hyperactivity-impulsivity.

Inattention symptoms include difficulty sustaining attention on a task, losing items necessary for tasks or activities, being easily distracted by external stimuli, not following instructions, and needing to be more mindful in daily activities.

Hyperactivity-impulsivity symptoms include difficulty sitting still or staying seated, excessive talking or interrupting others, fidgeting or squirming, acting without thinking about consequences, and difficulty waiting for one's turn.

It is essential to note that not all teenagers with ADHD exhibit all the symptoms and that the severity of symptoms can vary from person to person. The symptoms may also change as the teenager ages, with hyperactivity-impulsivity symptoms becoming less pronounced in adulthood.

Symptoms of ADHD will have a significant impact on a teenager's academic, social, and emotional development. You must be aware of these symptoms and provide appropriate support to help your son manage his symptoms and succeed.

- **DIAGNOSIS**

Diagnosing ADHD in teen boys can be complex, often involving multiple professionals such as pediatricians, psychologists, and psychiatrists. Several steps are typically involved in the diagnosis of ADHD.

The first step is a thorough medical and developmental history. The clinician will ask questions about your son's development, behavior, and academic performance. It's essential for you to provide detailed information about their child's behavior both at home and in other settings.

The next step is a physical exam, which may include neurological and hearing tests. This is done to rule out other medical conditions contributing to the teen's symptoms.

After the medical exam, the clinician may conduct behavioral assessments to evaluate the teen's attention, behavior, and emotional functioning. These assessments may include self-reporting questionnaires, interviews with the teen and family members, and observations of the teen in different settings.

To be diagnosed with ADHD, the teen must meet specific criteria outlined in the Diagnostic and Statistical Manual of Mental Disorders (DSM). These criteria include persistent and pervasive symptoms of inattention, hyperactivity, and impulsivity that interfere with daily functioning in two or more settings (such as home and school).

It's important to note that the diagnosis of ADHD is not a one-size-fits-all approach. The clinician will consider the teen's unique strengths and weaknesses, as well as their circumstances and environment. This is why working with a qualified, experienced professional who can provide a thorough and accurate diagnosis is essential.

Once a diagnosis has been made, the clinician will work with you and your son to develop an individualized treatment plan. This plan may include medication, behavioral therapy, educational accommodations, and other interventions tailored to the teen's needs.

You must be involved in the diagnosis process to ask questions and seek clarification. A proper diagnosis will help you better understand your teen behavior and provide them with the support and resources they need to succeed.

- **Principles of Parenting a Teen Boy with ADHD**

Parenting a teen boy with ADHD requires a unique approach considering the specific challenges of the condition. The following principles can help parents navigate these challenges:

1. **Education:** Educating yourself on ADHD and its symptoms is critical to effectively parenting a teen boy with this condition. Understanding how ADHD impacts your teen's behavior, emotions, and cognitive processes can help you develop effective strategies for managing their symptoms.

2. **Communication:** Effective communication is critical to successful parenting. It is vital to have open and honest communication with your teen about their condition, treatment options, and expectations. Encouraging your teen to express themselves and actively listening to their concerns and needs can

help you build a solid and trusting relationship.
3. **Consistency:** Consistency is essential for managing the symptoms of ADHD. Creating and sticking to a routine will help your son develop healthy habits and feel more secure. This includes maintaining consistent rules, expectations, and consequences.
4. **Positive reinforcement:** Positive reinforcement is a powerful tool for shaping your teen's behavior. Praising your son for his achievements and progress, rather than solely focusing on his shortcomings, will help build his confidence and self-esteem.
5. **Collaboration:** Collaborating with your teen's healthcare providers, educators, and other professionals can help ensure that your teen receives the appropriate treatment and support. Working together to create a comprehensive treatment plan will help address your teen's specific needs and goals.

By embracing these principles, you will effectively navigate the challenges of parenting a teen boy with ADHD and help them thrive.

• Assessment Questions to Determine if Your Teen Boy Has ADHD

Here are some assessment questions that will help you determine if your teen boy has ADHD:

1. Does your teen boy have difficulty paying attention or staying focused, especially in situations that are not interesting or stimulating to him?
2. Does your teen boy often make careless mistakes, lose things, or need help staying organized?
3. Does your teen boy struggle with following through on tasks or instructions, especially if they are repetitive or require sustained effort?
4. Does your teen boy have difficulty sitting still, fidgeting, squirming, or feeling restless?

5. Does your teen boy interrupt others frequently or have trouble waiting for his turn in conversations or activities?
6. Does your teen boy struggle with regulating his emotions, leading to outbursts of anger or frustration?
7. Does your teen boy have trouble sleeping or experience restless or interrupted sleep patterns?
8. Does your teen have difficulty paying attention to details and making careless mistakes?
9. Does your teen have trouble staying organized, even with reminders and support?
10. Does your teen struggle to complete tasks or follow through on instructions?
11. Does your teen seem not to listen when spoken to directly?
12. Does your teen often lose keys, phones, or school materials?
13. Does your teen avoid activities that require sustained mental effort?

14. Does your teen fidget or squirm when seated for an extended period?
15. Does your teen interrupt or intrude on others in conversation or activities?
16. Does your teen struggle with waiting his turn in conversations or games?
17. Does your teen have difficulty following rules or regulations at school or home?
18. Does your teen struggle with planning or organizing activities?
19. Does your teen often blurt out answers before the questions have been completed?
20. Does your teen frequently change activities or tasks before completing them?
21. Does your teen struggle with forgetfulness in daily activities?
22. Does your teen need help with long-term planning or setting goals?
23. Does your teen engage in risk-taking behaviors, like reckless driving or substance abuse?

24. Does your teen experience difficulty with social skills, like maintaining friendships or communicating effectively?
25. Does your teen struggle with emotional regulation or mood swings?
26. Does your teen have difficulty falling asleep or staying asleep?
27. Does your teen have a history of academic or behavioral problems at school?

Is your answer "yes" to several of these questions? In that case, it may indicate that your teen boy has ADHD and would benefit from further evaluation and support. It's important to consult a healthcare professional, for a formal diagnosis and treatment plan.

- **Things Your Teen Boy Wishes You Knew About ADHD**

Parenting a teen boy with ADHD can be challenging, but it's important to remember that your teen boy is also going through a tough time.

Here are some things your teen boy with ADHD will wish you knew:

1. ADHD is not a justification, but it does impact my behavior and emotions.
2. I'm not trying to be difficult or oppositional; my brain works differently than others.
3. It can be frustrating to forget or get distracted constantly, but I'm working on it.
4. Sometimes I need extra help or support to succeed.
5. I need to have structure and routine in my daily life.
6. I may struggle with self-esteem and self-worth because of my ADHD.
7. It's not helpful when you **compare me to other kids** or criticize me for my struggles with ADHD.
8. I'm not lazy, unmotivated, or unintelligent - I need extra support and understanding.
9. It can be overwhelming for me to manage my time and prioritize tasks.

10. I may struggle with impulsivity and making impulsive decisions.
11. I need to have clear expectations and consequences.
12. Sometimes I need reminders or prompts to stay on track.
13. Long periods of stillness can be challenging for me, especially if I'm not interested in what is going on.
14. I need extra time to process information or instructions.
15. I need to have breaks and downtime throughout the day.
16. I need help with social skills and making and maintaining friendships.
17. I need to have a supportive and understanding family environment.
18. Sometimes I need to take medication to manage my ADHD symptoms.
19. I need to have hobbies and interests that I enjoy and excel at.
20. I am more than my ADHD - I have strengths, talents, and abilities like anyone else.

In conclusion, this chapter has laid the foundation for understanding ADHD in teenage boys and the principles of parenting them. We have explored the symptoms and diagnosis of ADHD and provided you with assessment questions to help you determine if your teen boy has ADHD.

Additionally, we have shared insights into the things your teen boy with ADHD wishes you knew, which will help you develop a better understanding of their experiences and needs.

Moving forward, this book will delve deeper into the specific strategies, tools, and techniques that will help you support your teen boy with ADHD. We will explore various topics, such as creating a structured and organized environment, managing impulsivity and hyperactivity, improving communication and social skills, and supporting academic success.

Through practical exercises and interactive activities, you will learn how to implement these strategies effectively and support your teen boy's development. By following the principles outlined in this book, you can create a positive and supportive environment for your teen boy, where they can thrive and achieve their full potential.

Remember, parenting a teen boy with ADHD can be challenging, but it is also incredibly rewarding. By taking the time to understand his unique needs and providing him with the support he requires, you can help him navigate life's challenges with confidence and resilience. So let's continue this journey together and **unlock** your teen boy's potential.

Chapter 1
TAKING CHARGE OF ADHD IN YOUR TEEN BOY

It can be challenging to navigate the daily challenges and responsibilities that come with having an ADHD-affected teenage boy. Sometimes it is easy to feel helpless, overwhelmed, and even frustrated.

However, taking charge of your teen boy's ADHD is crucial in helping him lead a fulfilling life, despite his condition. This chapter aims to arm you with the tips and tricks you'll need to manage the ADHD in your adolescent boy.

From understanding the condition to developing effective communication skills, this chapter will empower you to participate in your teen's journey toward success actively. So, let's dive in and take charge of ADHD in your teen boy!

- **How to Take Charge of ADHD in Your Teen Boy**

Taking charge of ADHD in your teen boy can be challenging and overwhelming. Still, ensuring that your child receives the support and resources necessary to manage their condition effectively is essential. Here are some helpful hints to help you manage your teen boy's ADHD:

→ **EDUCATE YOURSELF**

As a parent of an ADHD teen boy, it is important to educate yourself about the condition. The more you know, the better equipped you will be to support your child. Here are some ways to educate yourself about ADHD:

1. **Read books and articles:** This book will give a very good knowledge about ADHD in your teen boy and how you will help them thrive.

2. **Attend workshops and seminars:** There are many workshops and seminars available that provide information on ADHD. These events are often led by experts in the field and can provide valuable information on how to support your child.

3. **Join support groups:** There are many support groups for parents of ADHD children. These groups can provide a safe space to share your experiences, ask questions, and learn from others who have similar experiences.

4. **Talk to professionals:** Speak to professionals such as pediatricians, psychologists, or psychiatrists who have experience with ADHD. They can provide valuable information and resources to help you better understand the condition.

5. **Use reliable online resources:** There are many online resources available that

provide information on ADHD. However, it is important to use reliable sources such as reputable medical websites, ADHD advocacy organizations, or government agencies.

By educating yourself about ADHD, you can better understand your teen boy's struggles and develop effective strategies to support him.

➔ **CREATING STRUCTURE AND ROUTINE**

It is extremely beneficial for your son to have structure and routine. It will help them to feel more organized, reduce their stress and anxiety, and improve their ability to focus and complete tasks.

Here are some tips on how to create structure and routine for your ADHD teen boy:

1. **Create a visual schedule:** Use a whiteboard or a calendar to create a visual schedule for your teen. This can help them to see what they need to do and when, which can reduce their anxiety and help them to stay on track.

2. **Set consistent routines:** Establish consistent routines for waking up, going to bed, mealtimes, and homework. This can help your teen to establish good habits and make it easier for them to transition between activities.

3. **Break tasks into smaller parts:** Help your teen to break tasks into smaller, more manageable parts. This can make it easier for them to focus and feel less overwhelmed.

4. **Use timers:** Set a timer to help your teen stay on track and focus on a specific task for a set amount of time. This can help

them to stay motivated and feel more in control of their time.

5. **Incorporate physical activity:** Encourage your teen to engage in physical activity, such as taking a walk or playing sports. This can help to reduce their stress and anxiety, and improve their ability to focus.

Remember, creating structure and routine takes time and patience. It may take some trial and error to find what works best for your teen. But with consistency and persistence, you can help your ADHD teen boy to thrive and succeed.

Encouraging healthy habits is crucial for every teenager's physical and mental well-being. However, it can be particularly challenging for a teen boy with ADHD. Here are some tips for parents to help their teen boy develop healthy habits:

1. **Set a regular sleep schedule:** Adequate sleep is essential for overall health and well-being. Encourage your teen to follow a consistent sleep schedule, even on weekends, to help regulate their circadian rhythm.

2. **Encourage regular exercise:** Exercise is a natural way to release excess energy and improve focus. Encourage your teen to engage in physical activities they enjoy, such as team sports, running, swimming, or martial arts.

3. **Promote healthy eating habits:** A balanced diet can help manage symptoms of ADHD and promote overall health. Encourage your teen to eat a variety of fruits, vegetables, lean proteins, and whole grains. Limit sugary and processed foods, which can worsen ADHD symptoms.

4. **Teach stress-management techniques:** Stress and anxiety can worsen ADHD

symptoms. Teach your teen relaxation techniques such as deep breathing, meditation, or yoga, to help manage stress.

5. **Limit screen time:** Excessive screen time can interfere with sleep and exacerbate ADHD symptoms. Encourage your teen to limit screen time and engage in other activities such as reading, playing board games, or spending time outdoors.

By promoting healthy habits, parents will help you with ADHD develop skills that will serve him well into adulthood. It is essential to establish healthy routines that prioritize sleep, exercise, healthy eating, stress management, and limited screen time.

➜ **Set clear expectations**
Setting clear expectations is crucial for any teenager, especially for those with ADHD. Here are some tips to help you set clear expectations for your ADHD teen boy:

1. **Be specific:** Vague expectations like "Do your best" or "Behave yourself" can be confusing for your ADHD teen. Instead, be specific about what you expect from them, such as completing homework by a certain time or following a set of house rules.

2. **Use visuals:** ADHD teens often respond well to visual aids. Consider creating a chore chart or schedule with pictures or symbols to help them understand what is expected of them.

3. **Be consistent:** Consistency is key when setting expectations for your ADHD teen. Stick to the rules you've established and be consistent in enforcing consequences.

4. **Provide positive reinforcement:** Praise your teen when they meet your expectations. Positive reinforcement can motivate them to continue meeting your expectations and build their confidence.

5. **Involve your teen in setting expectations:** Involve your teen in setting expectations, as this can help them take ownership of their behavior and feel more invested in meeting the expectations.

6. **Adjust expectations as needed:** Be open to adjusting your expectations if necessary. Your teen may struggle with certain expectations, and you may need to make adjustments to help them succeed.

Remember, setting clear expectations can be a process, and it may take some time for your ADHD teen boy to understand and meet your expectations consistently. Be patient, and continue to work with them to help them succeed.

➔ **Build a support team**

Building a support team for an ADHD teen boy is crucial for their success and well-being. Here are some steps to take:

1. **Identify potential team members:** Think about people in your teen's life who can support them in different ways. This could include family members, teachers, coaches, therapists, and friends.

2. **Communicate with team members:** Talk to each potential team member about your teen's diagnosis and what support they can offer. Be open and honest about your concerns and ask for their input and support.

3. **Create a plan:** Work with your team members to create a plan for supporting your teen. This plan should include specific strategies for managing ADHD symptoms, such as medication, therapy, and accommodations at school. It should also include ways that each team member

can provide support and help your teen reach his goals.

4. **Maintain regular communication:** Regular communication is essential for keeping your support team informed about your teen's progress and any changes in his symptoms or needs. Schedule regular check-ins and make sure everyone is on the same page.

5. **Monitor progress and adjust the plan if need be:** Keep track of your teen's progress and adjust the support plan as needed. Be open to feedback from your team members and be willing to make changes to ensure your teen is getting the support he needs.

Remember, building a support team is not a one-time event. It is an ongoing process that requires effort and commitment from everyone involved. But with the right support, your

ADHD teen boy can thrive and reach their full potential.

By taking charge of ADHD in your teen boy, you can help him lead a successful and fulfilling life while managing his symptoms effectively.

Ways to Transform Your Teen Boy with ADHD

Parenting a teen boy with ADHD can be challenging, but it can also be a fulfilling journey. As a parent, you possess the power to help your son transform his life for the better. Here are ways to do that:

1. Encourage regular exercise to help with impulsivity, hyperactivity, and inattention.
2. Create a structured routine that includes specific times for homework, meals, and other activities.
3. Set clear expectations and boundaries for behavior and consequences for breaking them.

4. Create a quiet and organized study space to minimize distractions.
5. Encourage your teen to use tools like calendars and planners to stay organized and on track.
6. Use positive reinforcement to motivate and encourage your teen's good behavior.
7. Help your teen develop healthy coping mechanisms for stress and anxiety.
8. Provide regular breaks during homework or study time to avoid burnout and frustration.
9. Limit screen time and encourage more productive activities like reading or outdoor activities.
10. Help your teen build a support network of friends, family, and professionals who can offer guidance and support.
11. Practice active listening and communicate with your teen in a non-judgmental and supportive way.
12. Encourage your teen to participate in extracurricular activities and hobbies that he enjoys.

13. Help your teen develop effective study habits, such as breaking down assignments into smaller tasks.
14. Use positive self-talk to help your teen build self-confidence and self-esteem.
15. Encourage your teen to take responsibility for their actions and decisions.
16. Provide consistent and regular feedback on their progress and growth.
17. Celebrate successes and milestones, no matter how small.
18. Encourage your teen to develop a growth mindset and see challenges as opportunities to learn and grow.
19. Provide regular opportunities for relaxation and self-care.
20. Model positive behavior and attitudes and strive to be a positive role model for your teen.
21. Encourage him to join a club or team that aligns with his interests. This can provide structure, socialization, and a sense of belonging.

22. Consider therapy or counseling to help your teen cope with ADHD and develop healthy coping strategies.
23. Help your teen boy build his self-esteem and confidence by focusing on his strengths and successes.
24. Set aside time each day for one-on-one bonding with your teen, such as sharing a meal or participating in a shared hobby.
25. Create a calming, distraction-free environment for homework and studying.
26. **Address co-occurring conditions:** Anxiety or depression are common co-morbidities among adolescents with ADHD. Addressing these conditions is essential for your teen's overall well-being.
27. Consider dietary changes, such as reducing sugar and processed foods, which may exacerbate ADHD symptoms.
28. Teach your teen time-management skills, such as breaking down tasks into smaller steps and prioritizing to-do lists.

29. Find positive role models for your teen who also have ADHD, such as successful entrepreneurs or athletes.
30. Celebrate small victories and progress, rather than focusing solely on setbacks or challenges.

By taking charge of your teen's ADHD, you can help them transform their lives and reach their full potential. Even though it won't always be simple, your patience and perseverance can make a difference.

- **Safe Care Tips for Your Teen Boy with ADHD**

When parenting a teen boy with ADHD, it's essential to prioritize his safety. The impulsivity and distractibility associated with ADHD can put them at risk of accidents or injury. Therefore, implementing safety measures in your home and everyday routines can significantly reduce the likelihood of such incidents.

Here are safe care tips for your teen boy with ADHD:
1. **Set up a safe home environment:** Remove any hazards, sharp objects, or dangerous tools from your home. Secure furniture to prevent tipping, and install safety gates and locks to prevent access to dangerous areas.
2. **Teach road safety:** Remind your teen boy to be mindful of traffic lights, signs, and pedestrian crossings. Ensure they know to look both ways before crossing the road and always wear reflective clothing when walking in the dark.
3. **Monitor medication use:** If your teen boy is taking medication for ADHD, ensure they take it as prescribed and store it safely out of their reach. Also, be aware of the side effects of the medication, and monitor any changes in behavior or mood.
4. **Encourage physical activity:** Regular exercise can help improve focus and attention in teens with ADHD. Encourage your teen boy to engage in physical

activities such as sports or outdoor games. Ensure they have proper safety equipment, such as helmets, when participating in sports.
5. **Establish routines:** Creating a routine can help your teen boy with ADHD feel more organized and in control. Please set a consistent schedule for sleep, meals, and homework, and ensure they stick to it.

By implementing these safe care tips, you will help your teen boy with ADHD to thrive in a safe and secure environment.

- **Prioritizing Yourself as a Parent of a Teen Boy with ADHD**

Being a parent of a teen boy with ADHD can be challenging, stressful, and overwhelming. As a parent, it's easy to put your child's needs before your own, but it's also essential to prioritize your own well-being. You can't take care of your child effectively if you don't care for yourself first.

Here are some ways to prioritize yourself as a parent of a teen boy with ADHD:

1. **Take breaks:** Make sure you're taking regular breaks throughout the day. It can be as simple as taking a few minutes to sit quietly, meditate, or walk outside. These breaks can help you recharge and reduce stress levels.
2. **Practice self-care:** Make time for self-care activities, such as exercise, reading, or spending time with friends. It's crucial to engage in activities that bring you joy and relaxation.
3. **Ask for help:** Consult family members, close friends, or a support group for parents of children with ADHD. Having a support network around you can make you feel less alone and give you emotional support.
4. **Establish boundaries:** To make sure you aren't taking on too much, it's crucial to establish boundaries with your child and

others. Be frank about your boundaries and let people know what they are.
5. **Get help:** Don't be afraid to seek professional help if you're struggling with the stress of parenting a teen boy with ADHD. Therapy, counseling, or medication can help you manage stress levels and improve your mental health.

Remember, taking care of yourself isn't selfish. It's necessary to be your best parent for your teen boy with ADHD.

- **Responding Appropriately to Different Behavioral Situations**

Parenting a teen boy with ADHD requires responding appropriately to different behavioral situations. Tips on how to handle specific situations:
1. **Hyperactivity:** When your teen boy is experiencing hyperactivity, it is important to provide outlets for physical activity. Encourage him to participate in sports or

other physical activities that allow him to release excess energy.
2. **Impulsivity:** Impulsivity can lead to poor decision-making and risky behaviors. As a parent, it's important to help your teen boy develop self-control. Encourage him to think before acting and provide consequences for impulsive behaviors.
3. **Inattention:** When your teen boy struggles with inattention, it's important to provide structure and routine. Ensure he has a designated study area and establishes regular routines for homework and chores.
4. **Anger and irritability:** Teenage boys with ADHD may have difficulty controlling their emotions, which can result in outbursts of annoyance and irritability. Assist your teen boy in learning coping mechanisms like deep breathing or taking a break to relax.
5. **Social situations:** ADHD makes social situations challenging for your son. Encourage your teen to participate in

social activities and respect his need for breaks and alone time.

Keep in mind that every adolescent with ADHD is different, so what works for one may not work for another. Be patient and willing to try different approaches to find the best for your teen boy.

- **Identifying Your Teen Boy's Triggers**

Identifying your teen boy's triggers is vital in managing his ADHD symptoms. Triggers are situations, events, or circumstances that can worsen your teen's ADHD symptoms. By identifying your teen's triggers, you can take steps to avoid or minimize them, which can help improve his overall functioning.

Triggers can vary widely from person to person. Still, some common triggers for teens with ADHD include stress, fatigue, boredom, sensory overload, and certain foods or drinks. It's essential to track when your teen's symptoms are at their worst and what is happening to help identify his specific triggers.

Once you have identified your teen's triggers, you can work with him to develop strategies for avoiding or managing them.

For example, if your teen's trigger is stress, you should teach him relaxation techniques like deep breathing or meditation. If his trigger is sensory overload, you should create a quiet, low-stimulation environment for him to work or study in.

It's also essential to communicate with your teen about his triggers and how they affect him. Encourage him to be aware of his motivations and to communicate with you when he feels overwhelmed or needs a break. By working together, you can develop a plan for managing his triggers and improving his overall well-being.

- **Handling Explosive Behavior Without Losing Control**

Parenting a teen boy with ADHD can be a challenging task, especially when it comes to handling explosive behavior. Explosive behavior is a common symptom of ADHD, and it can be difficult for parents to manage. However, it's important to remember that your teen boy's behavior does not reflect you as a parent, and there are strategies you can use to handle explosive behavior without losing control.

One of the first steps in managing explosive behavior is identifying triggers that can lead to outbursts, including things like frustration, fatigue, hunger, sensory overload, or overstimulation. Once you know what triggers your teen boy's explosive behavior, you can work on minimizing those triggers or finding alternative coping mechanisms for your teen boy.

It's also essential to set clear boundaries and consequences for explosive behavior. Let your teen boy know what behavior is acceptable, and be consistent in your approach; this may mean enforcing consequences like losing privileges or time-outs when your teen boy crosses the line. Remember to praise positive behavior and acknowledge when your teen boy tries to control their behavior.

When dealing with explosive behavior, staying calm and in control is essential. Avoid escalating the situation by shouting or becoming physically aggressive. Instead, try to remain calm and use a firm but gentle voice to communicate with your teen boy. Take a break if necessary, and return to the situation when you and your teen boy are calm and ready to talk.

Finally, seek support when you need it. Parenting a teen boy with ADHD can be overwhelming, and having a support system is essential; this may include talking to other parents who have been through similar experiences, seeking professional counseling, or joining a support group. Remember, you don't have to go through this alone.

- **Developing Social Awareness and Responsibility in Your Teen Boy**

You want your son to become socially responsible individuals who contribute positively to society. However, for parents of teenage boys with ADHD, developing social awareness and responsibility can be a challenging task.

Teen boys with ADHD often struggle with social skills, impulse control, and self-regulation, making it difficult to understand and respect social norms and rules. They may also have difficulty recognizing the impact of their actions on others, leading to social conflicts and challenges.

To help your teen boy with ADHD develop social awareness and responsibility, teaching him vital social skills such as empathy, communication, and conflict resolution is essential. Here are some tips to get started:

1. **Encourage Empathy:** Help your teen boy understand and identify emotions in themselves and others. Teach them to recognize body language and nonverbal cues to know how others feel. Practice having them put themselves in other people's shoes, and consider how their actions may affect others.
2. **Foster Communication Skills:** Communication skills are essential for developing healthy relationships and building social awareness. Encourage your teen boy to communicate clearly and effectively with others and to listen actively to what others are saying.
3. **Teach Conflict Resolution:** Conflict is a natural part of human interaction, but it can be challenging for those with ADHD. Help your teen boy develop the skills to resolve conflicts peacefully and to

negotiate solutions that work for all parties involved.
4. **Promote Social Involvement:** Social involvement can help teens with ADHD build social skills and connections. Encourage your teen to participate in group activities like clubs, sports, or community service.
5. **Model Positive Behavior:** As a parent, you play a critical role in modeling social awareness and responsibility. Make an effort to model positive behavior, such as empathy, communication, and conflict resolution, in your interactions with others.

By focusing on developing social awareness and responsibility in your teen boy with ADHD, you can help them build the skills to navigate social situations successfully and thrive in their relationships.

Chapter 2
HYPERACTIVITY

- **What Causes Hyperactivity in Teen Boys with Adhd?**

Hyperactivity in teen boys with ADHD is caused by a complex interaction of various factors. The exact cause of ADHD is not yet fully understood, but research suggests that genetic, environmental, and neurological factors may contribute to the development of the disorder.

In terms of genetics, studies have found that ADHD tends to run in families. This suggests that there may be a genetic component to the disorder. Environmental factors such as exposure to toxins, prenatal drug and alcohol exposure, and premature birth may also increase the risk of developing ADHD.

Neurological factors may also play a role in the development of hyperactivity in teen boys with ADHD. Studies have found differences in the structure and function of the brains of individuals with ADHD compared to those without the disorder. These differences may contribute to the hyperactivity and impulsivity seen in individuals with ADHD.

Furthermore, imbalances in the levels of certain neurotransmitters such as dopamine, norepinephrine, and serotonin may also contribute to the symptoms of hyperactivity in individuals with ADHD. These neurotransmitters are responsible for regulating attention, motivation, and behavior, and imbalances in their levels may disrupt these processes, leading to hyperactivity and impulsivity.

Overall, hyperactivity in teen boys with ADHD is likely caused by a complex interplay of genetic, environmental, and neurological factors, and a better understanding of these factors can help in the development of effective treatment strategies.

- **How does hyperactivity affect daily life?**

Hyperactivity in teen boys with ADHD can significantly affect their daily life in various ways. Some of the common effects include:

1. **Difficulty in staying focused and completing tasks:** Hyperactivity can make it challenging for teen boys with ADHD to stay focused on one task and complete it. They tend to be easily distracted by their surroundings, making it difficult to concentrate.
2. **Disruptive behavior:** Hyperactivity often leads to disruptive behavior in teen boys with ADHD. They may interrupt conversations, have difficulty waiting for their turn, and may have trouble following rules.
3. **Impulsivity:** Teen boys with ADHD may act impulsively, without thinking through the consequences of their actions. This can lead to poor decision-making and risky behaviors.
4. **Social difficulties**: Hyperactivity can also impact a teen boy's ability to socialize. They may struggle to control their behavior in social situations, leading to peer rejection and social isolation.
5. **Poor academic performance:** Hyperactivity makes it challenging for your son to focus and complete schoolwork. This can lead to poor

academic performance, which can further impact their self-esteem and motivation.

Overall, hyperactivity can significantly impact a teen boy's daily life, affecting their academic performance, social relationships, and overall well-being. It is essential to seek appropriate support and treatment to manage these symptoms effectively.

- **Physical symptoms:**
1. Restlessness and fidgeting
2. Difficulty sitting still or staying in one place
3. Excessive talking or interrupting others
4. Inability to engage in activities quietly
5. Constant movement, such as pacing or tapping fingers or feet
6. Difficulty waiting for one's turn in conversations or activities

- **Behavioral symptoms:**
1. Impulsivity and acting without thinking
2. Difficulty following rules or instructions
3. Disorganization and forgetfulness

4. Procrastination and difficulty starting or completing tasks
5. Risk-taking behaviors and poor judgment
6. Difficulty with time management and prioritizing tasks

- **Emotional symptoms:**
1. Frustration and irritability
2. Impatience and difficulty with delayed gratification
3. Low self-esteem and feelings of inadequacy
4. Difficulty regulating emotions, including anger and frustration
5. Anxiety and worry
6. Difficulty with social interactions, including making and keeping friends.

- **The diagnosis process**

The diagnosis process for hyperactivity in teen boys with ADHD usually involves the following steps:

1. **Initial assessment:** A primary care doctor or pediatrician may perform a preliminary evaluation of the teen's symptoms,

medical history, and family history. They may also conduct a physical exam to rule out other potential causes of the symptoms.
2. **Referral to a specialist:** If the doctor suspects ADHD, they may refer the teen to a mental health professional, such as a psychologist, psychiatrist, or neurologist, who specializes in diagnosing and treating ADHD.
3. **Diagnostic evaluation:** The specialist will typically perform a comprehensive evaluation that includes interviews with the teen and their parents or caregivers, standardized rating scales, and behavioral observations. They may also gather information from other sources, such as teachers or coaches, to get a complete picture of the teen's symptoms.
4. **Diagnosis:** Based on the evaluation, the specialist will determine whether the teen meets the diagnostic criteria for ADHD according to the DSM-5 (Diagnostic and Statistical Manual of Mental Disorders, Fifth Edition).
5. **Treatment planning:** If the teen is diagnosed with ADHD, the specialist will work with the family to develop a

treatment plan that may include medication, behavioral therapy, or a combination of both. They may also recommend additional evaluations or assessments to rule out other conditions that may co-occur with ADHD, such as anxiety or learning disorders.

- **Treatment options**

The most common treatment options for hyperactivity in teen boys with ADHD include:

1. **Medication:** Stimulant medications such as Ritalin and Adderall are commonly prescribed to help manage hyperactivity symptoms in ADHD. These medications work by increasing levels of neurotransmitters in the brain that regulate attention and behavior.
2. **Behavioral therapy:** Behavioral therapy can help teach teens with ADHD techniques for managing their hyperactivity and impulsivity. This can include techniques such as mindfulness, self-monitoring, and self-reinforcement.
3. **Parent training:** Parents of teens with ADHD can benefit from training in behavioral management techniques that

can help them better manage their child's hyperactivity. This can include strategies such as positive reinforcement, time-outs, and setting clear expectations and consequences.
4. **Classroom accommodations:** Teens with ADHD may benefit from accommodations in the classroom such as preferential seating, extra time on assignments and tests, and breaks as needed to help manage their hyperactivity.
5. **Exercise and physical activity:** Regular exercise and physical activity can help reduce hyperactivity symptoms in teens with ADHD. This can include activities such as team sports, martial arts, or simply going for a walk or bike ride.
6. **Dietary changes:** Some studies have suggested that dietary changes, such as reducing sugar and caffeine intake, can help reduce hyperactivity symptoms in teens with ADHD.

It is important to note that every individual with ADHD is unique and may require a personalized treatment plan that includes a combination of the above options or other interventions. It is important to work closely with a healthcare professional to determine the best treatment plan for each individual.

- **Alternative treatments and therapies**

There are various alternative treatments and therapies that can help manage hyperactivity in teen boys with ADHD. These include:

1. **Behavioral therapy:** This type of therapy involves teaching the teen how to change their behavior and develop coping mechanisms to manage their symptoms.
2. **Mindfulness meditation:** Meditation can help calm the mind and improve focus, reducing hyperactivity in some individuals.
3. **Exercise:** Regular physical activity can help burn off excess energy and improve focus and mood.
4. **Dietary changes:** Avoiding certain foods like sugar and processed foods and increasing consumption of healthy foods like fruits, vegetables, and lean protein can help improve symptoms.
5. **Supplements:** Certain supplements like omega-3 fatty acids and zinc have been found to be helpful in managing ADHD symptoms.

6. **Neurofeedback:** This is a type of therapy that uses technology to help the teen learn how to control their brain waves, improving focus and reducing hyperactivity.
7. **Art therapy:** Engaging in creative activities like painting or drawing can be therapeutic and calming, reducing hyperactivity.

It is important to note that these alternative treatments should not replace traditional medical treatment and should always be discussed with a healthcare professional.

- **Lifestyle Changes to Manage Hyperactivity**

→ **Diet and nutrition tips**
Making lifestyle changes can also be helpful in managing hyperactivity in teen boys with ADHD. One important aspect is diet and nutrition. Here are some tips to consider:

1. **Avoid processed foods:** Processed foods often contain high amounts of sugar, salt, and additives, which can exacerbate

hyperactivity symptoms. Instead, focus on fresh fruits, vegetables, and whole foods.
2. **Increase protein intake:** Protein helps to balance blood sugar levels, providing a steady supply of energy. Good sources of protein include lean meats, eggs, beans, and nuts.
3. **Reduce sugar and caffeine:** Both sugar and caffeine can worsen hyperactivity symptoms. Try to limit your teen's intake of sugary foods and drinks, and avoid caffeinated beverages like soda and energy drinks.
4. **Incorporate omega-3 fatty acids:** Omega-3 fatty acids have been shown to improve brain function and reduce symptoms of hyperactivity. Good sources include fatty fish, flaxseed, and walnuts.
5. **Consider supplements:** Certain supplements, such as magnesium, zinc, and iron, may also help to improve symptoms of hyperactivity. However, it's important to consult with a healthcare professional before adding any supplements to your teen's diet.

Remember that each teen's nutritional needs are unique, so it's important to work with a healthcare professional to develop a diet plan that is tailored to your teen's specific needs and preferences.

➔ **Exercise and physical activity recommendations**

Regular exercise and physical activity can help manage hyperactivity in teen boys with ADHD. Here are some recommendations:

1. Encourage at least 60 minutes of physical activity every day, such as playing sports, jogging, cycling, or swimming.
2. Incorporate activities that require focus and concentration, such as martial arts, yoga, or dance.
3. Choose activities that your teen boy enjoys and that are age-appropriate.
4. Create a routine or schedule for physical activity to establish consistency and structure.
5. Consider outdoor activities to provide exposure to sunlight and nature, which can help improve mood and attention.
6. Be sure to consult with your teen boy's healthcare provider before starting any new exercise program, especially if there are any medical concerns or conditions.

➜ **Sleep and relaxation strategies**

Getting enough quality sleep and relaxation is crucial for managing hyperactivity in teen boys with ADHD. Here are some tips:

1. Set a consistent bedtime and wake-up time, even on weekends.
2. Create a bedtime routine that promotes relaxation, such as taking a warm bath or reading a book.
3. Keep the bedroom dark, quiet, and cool to promote sleep.
4. Avoid stimulating activities, such as using electronic devices or watching TV, for at least an hour before bedtime.
5. Encourage relaxation techniques such as deep breathing, meditation, or yoga.
6. Make sure your teen boy has a comfortable and supportive mattress and pillow.
7. Limit caffeine intake, especially in the afternoon and evening.
8. Try to reduce stressors that can disrupt sleep, such as excess homework or too many extracurricular activities.

9. Avoid sleeping pills unless prescribed by a doctor.
10. Consider using white noise or a calming scent, such as lavender, to promote relaxation and improve sleep quality.

Chapter 3
IMPULSIVITY

Impulsivity is a behavioral trait characterized by acting without thinking, making decisions based on immediate gratification, and having difficulty inhibiting or delaying actions. In the context of ADHD, impulsivity refers to the tendency to act on impulse without considering the consequences or potential risks of one's actions.

- **Impulsivity as a symptom of ADHD**

Impulsivity is one of the three core symptoms of Attention Deficit Hyperactivity Disorder (ADHD), along with hyperactivity and inattention. Impulsivity refers to acting without forethought or considering the consequences of one's actions. It involves acting on impulse, being easily distracted, and having difficulty waiting for one's turn.

In teens with ADHD, impulsivity often manifests as interrupting others during conversations, blurting out answers before the question is complete, and having difficulty waiting in lines or taking turns during games.

In adults, impulsivity can lead to problems such as risky driving, impulsive spending, and difficulty maintaining relationships due to impulsive decisions and behaviors.

Impulsivity is thought to be caused by a dysfunction in the brain's prefrontal cortex, which is responsible for regulating attention, emotions, and decision-making. This dysfunction can result in a decreased ability to inhibit inappropriate behaviors and regulate emotional responses.

While impulsivity is a symptom of ADHD, it can also occur in individuals without ADHD. However, in those with ADHD, impulsivity tends to be more severe and pervasive, and it often co-occurs with the other core symptoms of ADHD. Effective treatment of ADHD typically involves a combination of medication, behavioral therapy, and environmental modifications.

- **Importance of understanding impulsivity in teen boys with ADHD**

This is crucial for several reasons:

1. **Treatment:** Impulsivity is one of the hallmark symptoms of ADHD, and it can significantly impact a teen's ability to function in school, at home, and in social situations. Understanding impulsivity can help identify the appropriate treatment options, such as medication, behavioral therapy, or a combination of both.
2. **Risk-taking behaviors:** Impulsivity can lead to risky behaviors such as substance abuse, reckless driving, or unsafe sexual practices. Understanding impulsivity can help parents and caregivers recognize potential risks and implement strategies to prevent them.
3. **Social relationships:** Impulsivity can interfere with a teen's ability to form and maintain healthy social relationships. It can lead to social isolation, rejection, and conflict with peers. Understanding impulsivity can help parents and caregivers provide appropriate guidance and support to improve social skills and relationships.
4. **Academic performance:** Impulsivity negatively impacts academic performance. Impulsive behaviors such as interrupting the teacher, being easily distracted, or not

following instructions can interfere with learning. Understanding impulsivity helps you to develop appropriate accommodations and strategies to support academic success.

Overall, understanding impulsivity in teen boys with ADHD is essential for improving their quality of life and helping them reach their full potential.

- **Impact of impulsivity on daily life**

The impact of impulsivity on daily life is significant for individuals with ADHD, especially for teen boys. Impulsive behavior can affect several areas of life, including social interactions, academic performance, and personal safety.

In terms of social interactions, impulsive behavior can lead to difficulty in forming and maintaining relationships. Impulsive individuals may interrupt others, speak without thinking, and struggle to take turns in conversations, which can be perceived as rude or insensitive. As a result, individuals with ADHD may find themselves isolated or excluded from social situations, which can lead to feelings of loneliness and depression.

Academically, impulsivity can affect a student's ability to focus and complete tasks. Impulsive behavior can lead to distractibility, difficulty with organization and planning, and a lack of impulse control, all of which can negatively impact academic performance. This can lead to low grades, poor attendance, and academic failure, which can have long-lasting consequences for future success.

In terms of personal safety, impulsivity can lead to risky behaviors. For example, a teen with ADHD may engage in impulsive driving behaviors, such as speeding or texting while driving, which can lead to accidents and injuries. Additionally, impulsivity can lead to substance abuse, sexual promiscuity, and other dangerous behaviors that can have negative consequences for physical and mental health.

Overall, understanding the impact of impulsivity on daily life is crucial for effectively managing ADHD symptoms. By recognizing how impulsivity affects social interactions, academic performance, and personal safety, individuals with ADHD can develop strategies to manage impulsive behavior and improve overall quality of life

- **Impact of impulsivity on daily life**

The impact of impulsivity on daily life can be significant for teen boys with ADHD. They may struggle to maintain friendships due to their impulsive behavior, such as interrupting others or being overly aggressive. In academic settings, impulsivity can result in poor grades, incomplete assignments, and difficulty following rules and instructions. In addition, impulsivity can lead to problems in the home environment, such as conflicts with parents or siblings.

- **Causes of Impulsivity in Teen Boys with ADHD**

1. Genetic factors
It plays a significant role in the development of ADHD, including impulsivity. Studies have shown that there is a strong heritability component to ADHD, with an estimated genetic contribution of 70-80%. This means that

individuals with a family history of ADHD are more likely to develop the disorder themselves.

Specific genes that have been linked to ADHD include those that are involved in regulating dopamine and norepinephrine levels in the brain. Dopamine is a neurotransmitter that is involved in reward processing, motivation, and impulse control, while norepinephrine is involved in attention and arousal.

One of the most well-studied genes associated with ADHD is the dopamine transporter gene (DAT1). Variations in this gene have been linked to alterations in dopamine transport and signaling, which can lead to increased impulsivity and other ADHD symptoms.

Other genes that have been implicated in ADHD include the dopamine receptor D4 gene (DRD4), the serotonin transporter gene (5-HTT), and the synaptosomal-associated protein 25 gene (SNAP-25).

→ **Environmental factors**
Environmental factors also play a significant role in the development of impulsivity in teen

boys with ADHD. These factors can include prenatal exposures, such as maternal smoking or exposure to alcohol or drugs during pregnancy, as well as postnatal factors such as early childhood stress, trauma, and adverse life events.

Research has also shown that parenting practices can affect the development of impulsivity in children with ADHD. Parents who are inconsistent with discipline, provide little supervision, or have high levels of conflict in the home can increase the likelihood of impulsivity in their children.

Additionally, social factors such as peer relationships, school environment, and community factors can also contribute to the development of impulsivity. For example, a lack of positive social support or exposure to violence in the community can increase the likelihood of impulsive behaviors.

Overall, the interaction of genetic and environmental factors likely contributes to the development of impulsivity in teen boys with ADHD. Understanding these factors can help inform interventions and treatments that target both the individual and their environment to promote better outcomes.

→ **Neurological factors**
It refers to abnormalities or dysfunctions in the brain that may contribute to impulsivity in teen boys with ADHD. Research suggests that differences in the prefrontal cortex, basal ganglia, and other brain regions that regulate cognitive control and emotion regulation may contribute to impulsivity in individuals with ADHD. Neurotransmitter imbalances, such as reduced dopamine levels, have also been associated with ADHD and impulsivity. Overall, neurological factors play an important role in the development and manifestation of impulsivity in teen boys with ADHD.

- **Managing Impulsivity in Teen Boys with ADHD**

→ **Medication**
One way to manage impulsivity in teen boys with ADHD is through medication. There are different types of medications that can help reduce impulsivity in individuals with ADHD, including stimulants such as methylphenidate

and amphetamines, and non-stimulants such as atomoxetine. These medications work by increasing the levels of certain neurotransmitters in the brain, which can improve attention, reduce hyperactivity, and control impulsive behaviors.

However, it is important to note that medication is not a cure for ADHD and may not work for everyone. It is also important to work closely with a healthcare professional to find the right medication and dosage that works for your son, as well as to monitor for potential side effects. Managing Impulsivity in Teen Boys with ADHD

➔ **Behavioral therapy**

This is a type of treatment that aims to modify problematic behaviors through various techniques such as positive reinforcement, rewards, and consequences. In the case of impulsivity in teen boys with ADHD, behavioral therapy can help teach them how to control their impulsive behaviors by rewarding them when they exhibit self-control and implementing consequences when they act impulsively.

→ Cognitive-behavioral therapy

Cognitive-behavioral therapy (CBT) is a form of talk therapy that focuses on the relationship between thoughts, feelings, and behaviors. CBT can be beneficial for teen boys with ADHD as it can help them identify and change negative thought patterns that may be contributing to their impulsivity. This type of therapy provides strategies for managing stress and improving overall emotional regulation.

→ Parent training

This program is effective in helping you learn how to manage your child's impulsive behaviors. These programs often teach parents behavioral techniques such as positive reinforcement and consequence implementation, as well as strategies for setting clear expectations and boundaries.

→ School-based interventions

School-based interventions for teen boys with ADHD may include accommodations such as preferential seating, extended time on assignments, and additional support from teachers or school counselors. School-based interventions can also involve teaching students coping strategies for managing their impulsivity in the classroom and social settings.

It's important to note that treatment for impulsivity in teen boys with ADHD is often multifaceted and may involve a combination of medication and various therapies. Additionally, each individual's treatment plan should be tailored to their specific needs and may require ongoing adjustments.

- **Strategies for Coping with Impulsivity**

Impulsivity can be challenging to manage, but there are several effective strategies that can help individuals cope with impulsivity:

➜ Mindfulness techniques
➜ Relaxation techniques
➜ Organization and planning strategies
➜ Exercise and physical activity
➜ Support groups

➔ Mindfulness techniques

Practicing mindfulness will help your son develop greater awareness of his thoughts and feelings, which helps him manage impulsive urges. Mindfulness techniques include deep breathing exercises, meditation, and body scan practices.

➔ Relaxation techniques

Relaxation techniques such as progressive muscle relaxation, yoga, and deep breathing exercises can help individuals reduce stress and anxiety, which can contribute to impulsive behaviors.

➔ Organization and planning strategies

Creating structure and routine in daily life can help individuals with impulsivity stay on track. This can include making to-do lists, using calendars or planners, and setting reminders.

➔ Exercise and physical activity

Regular exercise and physical activity can help individuals reduce stress, improve mood, and increase self-control, which can help manage impulsivity.

→ **Support groups**

Joining a support group or working with a therapist can provide individuals with a safe and supportive environment to discuss their struggles with impulsivity, gain insight, and learn coping strategies.

Overall, managing impulsivity involves developing greater self-awareness, building self-control skills, and finding effective strategies to cope with triggers and impulses. Different strategies may work better for different individuals, so it is important to experiment and find what works best for you.

Chapter 4
INATTENTION

- **Definition**

Inattention is a core symptom of ADHD (Attention Deficit Hyperactivity Disorder) and is characterized by difficulties in sustaining attention, being easily distracted, and having trouble organizing or completing tasks.

People with inattention problems struggle to follow through on instructions or finish schoolwork or household chores. They also have difficulty focusing on details and tend to make careless mistakes, often forgetful about routine activities, and may avoid tasks that require sustained mental effort.

These symptoms cause significant impairment in daily life and affect academic, occupational, and social functioning.

- **Importance of Addressing Inattention in Teen Boys with ADHD**

This is crucial for several reasons:

1. **Academic success:** Inattention can significantly impact academic performance, making it difficult for teens to complete homework and tests successfully. By addressing inattention, teens can improve their academic performance and increase their chances of succeeding in school.
2. **Social relationships:** Inattention can also affect teens' social relationships, leading to difficulties in making and maintaining friendships. Addressing inattention can help teens build stronger relationships with their peers.
3. **Emotional well-being:** Teens with ADHD experiences low self-esteem and negative emotions due to their inattention, which can lead to anxiety and depression. Addressing inattention can help improve emotional well-being and reduce the risk of developing mental health problems.
4. **Daily functioning:** Inattention can also impact daily functioning, making it difficult for teens to complete daily tasks, such as getting ready for school or work. By addressing inattention, teens can improve their ability to function in daily life and become more independent.

- **Signs and Symptoms**

Common signs and symptoms of inattention in ADHD include

1. **Difficulty sustaining attention:** Teen boys with ADHD may find it challenging to focus on tasks or activities for an extended period, especially if they are not enjoyable or interesting.
2. **Poor organization skills:** They may struggle with organizing and completing tasks, such as homework, chores, or projects.
3. **Forgetfulness:** They may forget or lose things needed for activities, such as school supplies, homework, or sports equipment.
4. **Careless mistakes:** They may make careless mistakes in schoolwork, exams, or other activities, despite knowing the correct answers.
5. **Difficulty with following instructions:** Teen boys with ADHD may have trouble following instructions or listening to others.
6. **Easily distracted:** They may get easily distracted by external stimuli, such as

noises, movements, or other people, making it challenging to focus on tasks.
7. **Lack of attention to detail:** They may struggle with paying attention to details and completing work accurately.
8. **Daydreaming:** They may appear to be "zoning out" or daydreaming, even in the middle of conversations or activities.
9. **Avoiding tasks:** They may try to avoid or delay tasks that require sustained attention or effort, such as schoolwork or household chores.

- **Differences between Inattention in ADHD and Typical Teenage Behaviors**

Inattention in ADHD is different from typical teenage behaviors in several ways. Some of the key differences include:

1. **Persistence:** Inattention in ADHD is persistent and consistent, whereas typical teenage behaviors may occur sporadically and in certain situations.
2. **Severity:** Inattention in ADHD is more severe than typical teenage behaviors and can significantly impact daily functioning and academic performance.

3. **Frequency:** Inattention in ADHD occurs more frequently and across multiple settings, whereas typical teenage behaviors may be limited to specific situations.
4. **Duration:** Inattention in ADHD lasts for a longer period of time than typical teenage behaviors, often persisting for at least six months.
5. **Interference:** Inattention in ADHD interferes with daily life and relationships, whereas typical teenage behaviors do not typically interfere with daily functioning.

It is important to note that while some inattention and distractibility are common in teenagers, those with ADHD often experience a more extreme and pervasive form of inattention that requires specific attention and management.

- **Factors Contributing to Inattention in Teen Boys with ADHD**

Inattention is a hallmark symptom of ADHD and can significantly impact the daily functioning and quality of life of teenage boys with this condition. The following are some of the factors that contribute to inattention in teen boys with ADHD:

1. **Neurobiological factors:** Research has shown that ADHD is associated with structural and functional abnormalities in the brain, particularly in the prefrontal cortex, which is involved in attention, working memory, and executive function. These differences in brain structure and function can contribute to inattention in individuals with ADHD.
2. **Genetics:** As discussed earlier, genetics plays a significant role in the development of ADHD. Individuals with a family history of ADHD are more likely to develop the disorder themselves, and specific genes that regulate dopamine and norepinephrine levels in the brain have been linked to ADHD symptoms, including inattention.
3. **Environmental factors:** While genetics plays a significant role in ADHD, environmental factors can also contribute to the development and severity of ADHD symptoms. Factors such as prenatal exposure to toxins, maternal stress, and early childhood experiences can all

contribute to inattention in individuals with ADHD.
4. **Co-occurring conditions:** Many individuals with ADHD also have co-occurring conditions, such as anxiety, depression, and learning disabilities, which can exacerbate inattention and make it more difficult to manage.
5. **Technology:** In today's society, technology is ubiquitous, and many teens spend a significant amount of time using electronic devices, such as smartphones and video games. Research has shown that excessive screen time can contribute to inattention and other ADHD symptoms.
6. **Sleep problems:** Sleep problems are common in individuals with ADHD and can contribute to inattention and other symptoms. Teenagers with ADHD may struggle with falling asleep, staying asleep, or having restful sleep, leading to daytime sleepiness and inattention.

Understanding these contributing factors will help you develop strategies to manage and reduce inattention in your son.

- **Behavioral Interventions**

These are an essential component of the management of inattention in teen boys with ADHD. These interventions are aimed at modifying behaviors and increasing desirable behaviors while decreasing undesirable behaviors. The following are some of the behavioral interventions used in managing inattention in teen boys with ADHD.

1. **Positive Reinforcement:** Positive reinforcement involves rewarding a child for appropriate behavior. In the case of inattention in teen boys with ADHD, positive reinforcement can be used to reinforce desirable behaviors, such as paying attention, completing tasks, and following instructions. The rewards can be in the form of praise, privileges, or tangible rewards, such as toys or money.
2. **Token Economy:** A token economy is a reward system that uses tokens or points that can be exchanged for rewards. Tokens can be given to a teen boy with ADHD for appropriate behavior, and these tokens can be exchanged for privileges or tangible rewards. Token economies are effective in

increasing desirable behaviors and reducing undesirable behaviors.
3. **Time Management Techniques:** Time management techniques involve teaching a teen boy with ADHD how to manage their time effectively. This includes setting goals, prioritizing tasks, and breaking down tasks into manageable steps. Time management techniques also involve teaching the teen boy how to use a planner or a calendar to schedule their tasks and activities.
4. **Environmental Modifications:** Environmental modifications involve changing the environment to reduce distractions and increase the likelihood of the teen boy with ADHD paying attention. Examples of environmental modifications include minimizing noise levels, reducing visual distractions, and using color-coding to organize materials and tasks.

In conclusion, behavioral interventions such as positive reinforcement, token economy, time management techniques, and environmental modifications can be used to manage inattention in teen boys with ADHD.

These interventions are effective in increasing desirable behaviors and reducing undesirable behaviors, leading to improved academic and social outcomes for your son.

- **Medication Management**

This is an essential aspect of treating ADHD, particularly in teenage boys. Medications are often prescribed to help manage the symptoms of ADHD, including inattention, hyperactivity, and impulsivity. The following is an overview of medication management in the treatment of ADHD.

➔ Types of Medications for ADHD

There are two main types of medications used to treat ADHD: stimulants and non-stimulants.

Stimulants are the most commonly prescribed medications for ADHD. They work by increasing the levels of dopamine and norepinephrine in the brain, which helps to improve attention and reduce impulsivity. Examples of stimulants include methylphenidate (Ritalin, Concerta), dextroamphetamine (Dexedrine), and mixed amphetamine salts (Adderall).

Non-stimulant medications are typically prescribed if stimulants do not work or cause significant side effects. Non-stimulants work by increasing the levels of norepinephrine in the brain. Examples of non-stimulants include atomoxetine (Strattera), guanfacine (Tenex), and clonidine (Kapvay).

→ **Side Effects and Risks**

While medication can be effective in managing ADHD symptoms, there are potential side effects and risks to consider. Common side effects of stimulant medications include decreased appetite, sleep problems, and irritability. Some individuals may also experience headaches, stomachaches, or increased heart rate. Non-stimulant medications can cause side effects such as nausea, dizziness, and fatigue.

There is also a risk of abuse and addiction with stimulant medications. Individuals who misuse or abuse stimulant medications may experience increased heart rate, high blood pressure, and potentially dangerous heart rhythms.

- **Medication Compliance**

Medication compliance is crucial for managing ADHD symptoms effectively. It is important for individuals with ADHD to take their medication consistently and as prescribed by their healthcare provider. This may involve taking medication at specific times of the day or adjusting the dosage based on individual needs.

It is also important for you to monitor medication compliance and make adjustments as needed. If medication is not working or causing significant side effects, it is necessary to switch to a different medication or adjust the dosage.

In conclusion, medication management is an important aspect of treating ADHD in teenage boys. While there are potential risks and side effects, medication can be effective in managing symptoms and improving overall quality of life. Close monitoring of medication compliance and side effects is necessary for successful treatment.

- **Psychotherapy**

Psychotherapy is a type of treatment for ADHD that aims to help individuals better understand and manage their symptoms. There are several types of psychotherapy that can be used to treat ADHD, including cognitive-behavioral therapy (CBT), mindfulness-based therapies, and family therapy.

Cognitive-Behavioral Therapy (CBT)

1. Cognitive-behavioral therapy (CBT) is a type of therapy that focuses on changing negative thought patterns and behaviors. In the case of ADHD, CBT can help individuals identify and challenge negative thoughts and beliefs about themselves, as well as develop coping strategies for managing symptoms. CBT for ADHD may also include strategies for improving time management, organization, and study skills.

Mindfulness-Based Therapies

2. Mindfulness-based therapies, such as mindfulness-based stress reduction (MBSR) and mindfulness-based cognitive therapy (MBCT), are designed to help individuals develop awareness and acceptance of their thoughts, emotions, and physical sensations.

Mindfulness-based therapies can be beneficial for individuals with ADHD by helping them develop greater self-awareness and emotional regulation skills, as well as reducing stress and anxiety.

Family Therapy

3. Family therapy involves working with the family as a whole to address issues related to ADHD. Family therapy can help parents better understand their child's symptoms and develop strategies for managing them, as well as improve communication and problem-solving skills within the family. Family therapy may also address any issues related to parenting and family dynamics that may be contributing to the child's symptoms.

It is important to note that psychotherapy should not be used as a substitute for medication management, as medication has been shown to be effective in reducing symptoms of ADHD. However, psychotherapy can be used in combination with medication to provide a more comprehensive approach to treating ADHD.

Additionally, psychotherapy can provide individuals with skills and strategies for managing their symptoms even when medication is not an option.

- **Educational Support**

Educational support is an essential component of managing inattention in teen boys with ADHD. Here are some of the common educational support strategies:

1. **Individualized Education Programs (IEPs):** IEPs are plans developed by a team of educators, parents, and other specialists to address the unique needs of a student with disabilities, including ADHD. IEPs typically include specific goals, accommodations, and modifications to help students with ADHD succeed academically.
2. **504 Plans:** A 504 plan is a written plan that outlines the accommodations and modifications that a student with a disability, including ADHD, requires to access and participate in their education. It is developed by a team of educators and parents, and it is designed to provide equal educational opportunities for students with disabilities.

3. Tutoring and Academic Coaching: Tutoring and academic coaching can be beneficial for students with ADHD who struggle with inattention and organization. These programs offer additional support and guidance to help students stay on track and manage their academic workload.

It is important to note that educational support strategies should be tailored to the individual needs of the student. Students with ADHD may require different types of support depending on their specific symptoms and challenges.

Effective educational support for students with ADHD involves collaboration between you, educators, and other professionals to create a comprehensive plan that addresses the student's academic and behavioral needs. Regular communication and monitoring of the student's progress are also critical components of successful educational support.

- **Tips for Parenting a Teen Boy with Inattention in ADHD**

Parenting a teen boy with inattention in ADHD can be challenging, but there are strategies parents can use to support their child's success. Here are some tips for parenting a teen boy with inattention in ADHD:

1. **Developing a Positive Parent-Child Relationship**: Establishing a positive and supportive relationship with your teen is important in managing his ADHD symptoms. This can include active listening, offering praise and encouragement, spending quality time together, and being involved in their interests and activities.
2. **Effective Communication Strategies:** Clear and effective communication can help prevent misunderstandings and conflicts. Some strategies to use include active listening, using "I" statements, avoiding criticism, and acknowledging your child's feelings.
3. **Setting Realistic Expectations and Goals:** Teens with ADHD may have difficulty with organization and time management, and may struggle to complete tasks or follow through on commitments. Setting realistic expectations and breaking tasks down into

smaller steps can help your teen feel less overwhelmed and more successful.
4. **Self-Care for Parents:** Taking care of yourself as a parent is essential to managing your own stress and being able to provide effective support for your child. This can include prioritizing self-care activities such as exercise, meditation, or hobbies, seeking support from family and friends, and seeking professional help if needed.
5. **Seeking Professional Help:** Consider seeking help from a mental health professional who has experience working with teens with ADHD. They can provide additional support and guidance on effective parenting strategies, medication management, and educational support.

Conclusion

In conclusion, inattention in teen boys with ADHD is a complex issue that requires a multifaceted approach to address effectively. By understanding the common signs and symptoms of inattention, the factors contributing to it, and the available interventions, you will be able to make informed decisions to help your son thrive.

Whether through medication management, behavioral interventions, psychotherapy, or educational support, there are a variety of tools and strategies available to support these young individuals. It is essential to prioritize developing positive parent-child relationships, effective communication, setting realistic expectations and goals, and self-care for your son.

By doing so, you will empower your son to overcome the challenges of inattention and reach his full potential. Let us work together to create a supportive environment that promotes the success and well-being of our teen boys with ADHD.

Chapter 5

STRATEGIES FOR DAILY LIFE

Welcome to the chapter on Strategies for Daily Life. Parenting a teen boy with ADHD can be challenging, but with the right strategies and tools, you can help your child manage their symptoms and lead a successful life. In this chapter, we'll explore a variety of practical tips and techniques you can implement in your teen's daily life to help them stay organized, focused, and productive. From creating a structured routine to practicing mindfulness, these strategies support your teen's unique needs and help them thrive. Let's get started!

- **Creating Routines and Schedules that Work**

Creating routines and schedules is an essential strategy in managing daily life for a teen boy with ADHD. Having a predictable structure to the day helps reduce stress and anxiety while improving focus and productivity. As a parent, you can work with your teen boy to create a routine and schedule that suits their needs, considering their ADHD symptoms and medication schedule.

One way to create a routine is by breaking the day into manageable chunks. You can use a whiteboard or planner to map out a schedule that includes regular meals, homework time, social activities, and exercise. Small breaks between activities can also help your teen boy recharge and refocus.

It's essential to be flexible and adjust the routine while maintaining consistency. Encourage your teen boy to take ownership of their way and have them actively participate in the process. With time and practice, creating routines and schedules will become a valuable habit that benefits you and your teen boy.

- **Managing Time and Priorities**

Managing time and priorities is crucial for individuals with ADHD. It can be particularly challenging for teenagers still developing their executive functioning skills. As a parent, you will help your teen boy with ADHD by teaching him effective time management techniques; this includes creating a schedule or routine that works for him, breaking tasks into smaller, more manageable pieces, and setting achievable goals.

One effective strategy for managing time and priorities is to use a planner or calendar; this allows your teen to keep track of upcoming assignments, appointments, and deadlines. You can work with your teen to establish a routine for updating the planner, such as checking it at the same time each day. Encouraging your teen to use reminders and alarms can also be helpful.

In addition to using a planner, you can help your teen prioritize tasks by breaking them down into smaller, more manageable steps; this will help him feel less overwhelmed and more in control. Encourage your teen to tackle the most important tasks and take breaks to avoid burnout.

Finally, it's essential to recognize that managing time and priorities is a continual process of trial and error. Be patient with your teen and encourage him to experiment with different strategies to find the best for him.

- **Helping Your Teen Boy Stay Organized**

As a parent of a teen boy with ADHD, helping him stay organized can be a significant challenge. ADHD often makes keeping track of schedules, deadlines, and belongings challenging. However, there are strategies you can use to help your teen boy stay organized and on top of things.

One effective strategy is establishing a designated place for your teen boy's belongings. For example, a designated area for backpacks, jackets, and shoes can help reduce the risk of losing essential items. Encouraging your teen boy to keep a tidy and organized space will be beneficial.

Another helpful strategy is to create a visual schedule or planner to help your teen boy keep track of his daily tasks, appointments, and deadlines. Consider using color-coded labels or symbols to make the planner more engaging and easier to understand.

Technology is also a valuable tool for staying organized. Numerous apps and digital tools will help your teen boy manage his time and keep track of his schedule. For example, setting reminders and alerts on a smartphone or tablet will be a great way to help your teen boy remember important tasks and deadlines.

Overall, helping your teen boy stay organized requires patience and creativity. By using a combination of strategies that work for your family, you can help your teen boy manage his ADHD symptoms and thrive in daily life.

- **Promoting Healthy Habits for Success**

Promoting healthy habits is essential for the success of any individual, especially for a teenager with ADHD. Teens with ADHD often struggle with managing their emotions, staying focused, and following through with tasks. Establishing healthy habits can help them to address these challenges better.

One essential habit is getting enough sleep. Getting enough sleep is crucial for mental and physical health. Lack of sleep can worsen ADHD symptoms, leading to difficulty focusing and irritability. To promote better sleep, establish a consistent bedtime routine and make sure your teen avoids caffeine and screens before bed.

Another critical habit is exercise. Exercise can help improve focus and mood, reduce stress and anxiety, and boost overall health. Encourage your teen to engage in regular physical activity, such as sports or a daily walk or run.

Healthy eating is also crucial for teens with ADHD. A well-balanced diet with plenty of fruits, vegetables, whole grains, and protein can help improve focus and reduce hyperactivity.

Avoid sugary, processed foods, and encourage your teen to eat regular daily meals.

Finally, practicing mindfulness and stress-reducing techniques such as meditation or deep breathing exercises can help your teen manage their emotions and reduce stress levels.

By promoting healthy habits, you will help your teen manage his ADHD symptoms and set him up for success in his daily life.

- **Improving Sleep Habits**

Improving sleep habits is essential to helping your teen boy with ADHD manage their symptoms and thrive daily. Sleep plays a crucial role in regulating mood, attention, and behavior. A lack of quality sleep can exacerbate ADHD symptoms.

To improve your teen's sleep habits, encourage him to establish a regular sleep schedule and stick to it as much as possible, even on weekends. A consistent bedtime and wake-up time help regulate the body's internal clock and promote quality sleep.

Additionally, a bedtime routine can signal the body that it is time to wind down and prepare for sleep. The routine could involve taking a warm bath or shower, reading a book, or listening to calming messages.

It's also essential to create a sleep-conducive environment. Make sure the bedroom is quiet, dark, and at a comfortable temperature. Encourage your teen to avoid using electronic devices in the bedroom, as the blue light emitted by screens can disrupt sleep.

If your teen struggles with falling asleep, consider relaxation techniques such as deep breathing, visualization, or progressive muscle relaxation. You may also consult a healthcare professional for further guidance on improving your teen's sleep habits.

- **Navigating Social Situations and Friendships**

Navigating social situations and friendships can be challenging for many teenagers, especially those with ADHD. Teenagers with ADHD may struggle with impulsivity, poor social skills, and difficulty reading social cues, making it hard to develop and maintain friendships. As a parent, there are several ways you can support your teen boy with ADHD in navigating social situations and building positive relationships with peers.

First, it's essential to help your teen boy develop social skills; this may include coaching him on how to start and maintain a conversation, read social cues, and manage his impulsivity in social situations. You can also encourage your teen to participate in social activities that align with his interests, such as joining a sports team or club.

It's also important to teach your teen boy with ADHD about appropriate social boundaries and how to communicate his needs effectively. For example, if your teen feels overwhelmed in a social situation, he may need to excuse himself and take a break. Encouraging your teen to communicate his needs clearly and respectfully will help him build positive relationships with others.

Another critical aspect of navigating social situations is helping your teen boy develop empathy and perspective-taking skills; this can involve talking with your teen about how others might feel in different social situations and encouraging him to consider different perspectives; this can help your teen better understand others and build stronger, more empathetic relationships.

Finally, monitoring your teen's social interactions and providing guidance and support as needed is essential; this may involve helping your teen identify and avoid toxic or harmful social situations and giving guidance on how to respond to conflict or other challenging situations. With your support and advice, your teen boy with ADHD can navigate social

situations and develop positive, supportive relationships with peers.
- **Helping Your Teen Boy Manage Screen Time**

In today's world, screen time has become an integral part of our daily lives. While it has advantages, it can also pose challenges, especially for teens with ADHD. Overstimulation and the constant need for instant gratification can lead to a lack of focus and decreased productivity. Therefore, it's essential to help your teen boy manage his screen time effectively.

Firstly, it's essential to set limits on the amount of time your teen spends on screens. Establish clear rules around using devices during meal times, homework, and other essential activities. Encourage your teen to take frequent breaks to avoid burnout and eye strain.

Secondly, monitor the type of content your teen is engaging with online. Screen time should be purposeful and beneficial. Encourage your teen to engage in activities that promote learning and growth, such as educational videos or interactive games that stimulate the brain.

Thirdly, model healthy screen habits yourself. Your teen boy is likely to follow your example, so ensure you practice what you preach. Try to limit your screen time and demonstrate to your teen that there are other enjoyable activities besides staring at a screen.

Lastly, encourage your teen to engage in other activities that do not involve screens, such as reading, playing sports, or spending time outdoors. Encourage your teen to develop hobbies and interests that allow him to explore and learn new things. By doing so, you'll be helping your teen develop a well-rounded personality while managing his screen time effectively.

Chapter 6
ACADEMIC SUCCESS

Academic success is essential to your teen boy's life and can be particularly challenging for those with ADHD. However, your teen boy can thrive academically with the right strategies, tools, and support. This chapter will provide practical and effective tips to help your teen boy achieve academic success, whether in middle school, high school, or college.

From developing good study habits and time management skills to working with teachers and managing accommodations, this chapter will equip you with the knowledge and resources to support your teen boy's academic growth and achievement.

- **Supporting Learning at Home**

Supporting learning at home is essential for academic success for any child, and it is essential for a teen boy with ADHD. As a parent, you can help create a positive and conducive learning environment at home; this can be achieved by establishing a designated study area for your teen boy, free from distractions such as TV and video games. Ensure the study area is well-lit, has a comfortable chair, and a desk with adequate space for books, computers, and other school supplies.

You will also help your teen boy develop good study habits by setting up a regular study routine with scheduled breaks. Breaks can be used as a reward for finishing a task or as a chance to recharge and refocus. Encourage your teen boy to take advantage of the break time by relaxing, such as going for a walk, playing a game, or engaging in physical activity.

Another way to support learning at home is by fostering good communication with your teen boy's teachers. Regularly check in with teachers to understand how your teen boy is performing academically and behaviorally in class; this will help you identify any challenges your teen boy may be facing and work with teachers to develop strategies for addressing them.

Ultimately, by providing a supportive learning environment at home, establishing a regular study routine, and fostering open communication with teachers, you can help your teen boy with ADHD achieve academic success.

- **Strategies for Success at School**

Helping your teen boy with ADHD achieve academic success can be a challenge. Still, it's possible with the right strategies in place. This chapter focuses on various approaches you must take to support your teen's academic achievement.

From working with teachers and school administrators to developing study skills and organization techniques, you'll learn how to create a supportive environment that helps his academic pursuits academically. We'll also explore ways to help your teen manage their ADHD symptoms in the classroom, such as reducing distractions and promoting healthy habits for focus and attention. By prioritizing your teen's academic success and implementing these strategies, you can help set them on a path to achieving success.

How to Create A Supportive Environment that Helps your Son

Creating a supportive environment for your ADHD teen son's academic pursuits is crucial for fostering success and minimizing challenges.

Understanding ADHD: Begin by educating yourself about ADHD, including its symptoms, challenges, and strengths. Understanding how ADHD impacts your teen's learning style and behavior is essential for providing effective support.

Establish Clear Expectations: Set clear, realistic academic expectations for your teen son. Break down tasks into manageable steps and establish routines to help him stay organized and focused.

Create a Distraction-Free Study Space: Designate a quiet, clutter-free study area where your teen can concentrate on his schoolwork without distractions. Remove electronic devices and other potential distractions to help him stay focused.

Use Visual Aids and Timers: Visual aids such as calendars, to-do lists, and schedules can help your teen son better manage his time and tasks. Utilize timers to break study sessions into manageable chunks and provide regular breaks to prevent overwhelm.

Encourage Regular Exercise and Healthy Habits: Physical activity is essential for managing ADHD symptoms and improving focus. Encourage your teen son to engage in regular exercise and prioritize healthy habits such as adequate sleep, nutritious diet, and hydration.

Implement Organization Strategies: Help your teen son develop organizational skills by teaching him how to use planners, checklists, and other organizational tools. Encourage him to break tasks into smaller steps and prioritize his workload.

Provide Emotional Support: Be empathetic and supportive of your teen son's struggles with ADHD. Encourage open communication and validate his feelings. Offer praise and encouragement for his efforts, regardless of the outcome.

Collaborate with Teachers and School Personnel: Establish open communication with your teen son's teachers and school personnel. Work together to develop an Individualized Education Program (IEP) or 504 Plan that outlines accommodations and supports tailored to his needs.

Explore Learning Strategies: Help your teen son discover effective learning strategies that work for him. This may include using mnemonic devices, breaking information into smaller chunks, or utilizing multi-sensory learning techniques.

Celebrate Achievements: Celebrate your teen son's academic achievements, no matter how small. Recognize his progress and efforts, and offer positive reinforcement to boost his confidence and motivation.

By implementing these strategies and creating a supportive environment at home, you can help your ADHD teen son thrive academically and reach his full potential. Remember to remain patient, flexible, and understanding as you navigate the challenges together.

Ways to help your teen manage his ADHD symptoms in the classroom

Helping your teen manage their ADHD symptoms in the classroom is crucial for their academic success and overall well-being. Here are several effective strategies to support your teen in this endeavor:

Open Communication: Encourage your teen to communicate openly with their teachers about their ADHD and any specific challenges they may face in the classroom. This allows teachers to provide appropriate accommodations and support.

Establish Routines: Help your teen establish daily routines for school tasks such as organizing their backpack, planning homework assignments, and preparing for exams. Consistent routines can help minimize distractions and improve focus.

Use Visual Aids: Visual aids such as color-coded notebooks, calendars, and task lists can help your teen stay organized and on track with assignments and deadlines. Encourage them to use visual reminders to prioritize tasks and manage their time effectively.

Break Tasks into Manageable Steps: Teach your teen to break down larger tasks or assignments into smaller, more manageable steps. This can make tasks feel less overwhelming and help them stay focused and motivated.

Provide Regular Breaks: Allow your teen to take regular breaks during periods of focused work. Short breaks can help prevent mental fatigue and improve attention span. Encourage them to engage in brief physical activities or relaxation techniques during breaks.

Seat Placement: Work with your teen's teacher to arrange seating in the classroom that minimizes distractions and maximizes focus. Consider placing your teen closer to the teacher's desk or away from windows, doors, or other sources of distraction.

Utilize Assistive Technology: Explore the use of assistive technology tools such as text-to-speech software, speech-to-text apps, or graphic organizers to help your teen with note-taking, organization, and comprehension of written material.

Implement Behavior Contracts: Consider implementing a behavior contract with your teen and their teacher to outline specific goals, expectations, and consequences for behavior in the classroom. This can help reinforce positive behaviors and encourage accountability.

Encourage Self-Advocacy: Teach your teen to advocate for themselves by asking for help when needed, requesting accommodations, or communicating their needs to teachers and classmates in a respectful manner.

Promote Healthy Lifestyle Habits: Encourage your teen to prioritize healthy lifestyle habits such as regular exercise, balanced nutrition, adequate sleep, and stress management techniques. A healthy lifestyle can help improve focus, attention, and overall well-being.

Provide Positive Reinforcement: Recognize and praise your teen's efforts and accomplishments in managing their ADHD symptoms in the classroom. Positive reinforcement can boost their confidence and motivation to continue using effective strategies.

By implementing these strategies and working collaboratively with your teen, their teachers, and other school personnel, you can help your teen effectively manage their ADHD symptoms in the classroom and thrive academically. Remember to remain patient, supportive, and understanding as your teen navigates the challenges of ADHD in an educational setting.

- **Managing Home Assignments**

Managing homework and assignments can be a significant challenge for teens with ADHD, and it can also be a primary source of stress for parents. However, there are many strategies you can use to help your teen boy manage homework and assignments more effectively.

First, it's essential to establish a consistent routine for homework and assignments; this might involve setting homework time each day and establishing and establishing a fixed location where your teen can work. Creating a structured plan for each assignment is essential, breaking it down into smaller tasks that can be tackled individually.

In addition to establishing a routine and creating a plan, it can be helpful to provide your teen with a quiet and distraction-free workspace and set clear expectations around completing assignments. You may also need to provide additional support, such as checking in regularly to see how your teen is progressing and helping to break down complex assignments into smaller, more manageable parts.

Other strategies that will be helpful include:
- Minimizing distractions during homework time.
- Providing breaks when needed.
- Using tools like timers or alarms to help your teen stay on track.

Consider exploring assistive technology or other tools to help your teen with reading, writing, or other academic tasks.

Ultimately, the key to managing homework and assignments with ADHD is to be patient, consistent, and supportive. With the right strategies, your teen can succeed academically and build the skills they need to thrive in school and beyond.

- **Preparing for Tests and Exams**

Preparing for tests and exams can be a challenging task for any student. Still, it can be particularly daunting for a teen boy with ADHD. The stress and pressure of exams can make it difficult for him to focus and concentrate, leading to poor performance and lower grades.

To help your teen boy prepare for tests and exams, creating a study plan that works for him is essential. Here are some strategies to consider:

1. **Break-up study sessions:** Encourage your teen boy to study in shorter sessions

with breaks in between; this can help him to stay focused and avoid burnout.
2. **Create a study schedule:** Help your teen boy create a study schedule that outlines what he needs to study and when; this can help him to stay on track and avoid last-minute cramming.
3. **Use visual aids:** Visual aids, such as diagrams, mind maps, and flashcards, can be a helpful way for your teen boy to memorize key concepts and information.
4. **Encourage active learning:** Encourage your teen boy to actively engage with the material he is studying; this could involve taking notes, summarizing key points, or discussing the material with someone else.
5. **Practice self-care:** Encourage your teen boy to practice self-care during the exam period; this could involve getting enough sleep, eating well, and taking breaks to exercise or engage in other relaxing activities.
6. **Speak to teachers:** If your teen boy struggles with exam preparation, speak to

his teachers or guidance counselor. They can offer additional support or resources.

Remember, every student is different, and what works for one student may not work for another. Experiment with different strategies and techniques until you find what works best for your teen boy.

- **Navigating the IEP and 504 Process**

Navigating the Individualized Education Program (IEP) and Section 504 Plan process can be a challenging experience for parents of teens with ADHD. However, it is essential to understand and utilize these programs to ensure that your teen boy receives the support and accommodations necessary for academic success.

The IEP is a legal document that outlines the individualized education plan for students with disabilities, including ADHD. It includes information on the student's needs, goals, and accommodations required for success in the classroom. The plan is developed in collaboration with the student, parents, teachers, and other relevant professionals, such as school psychologists or educational therapists.

On the other hand, Section 504 is a civil rights law that ensures students with disabilities, including ADHD, have equal access to education. The plan provides accommodations, modifications, and related services to help students with ADHD meet their academic needs. Navigating the IEP and 504 processes involves several steps, including identifying the need for accommodations, gathering documentation, attending meetings, and advocating for your teen boy's needs. It is essential to keep detailed records of your teen boy's progress, including academic reports, teacher feedback, and behavior logs. These records can help you and your teen's educators identify areas for additional support or accommodations.

When attending IEP and 504 meetings, come prepared with questions and concerns, and be ready to discuss your teen's strengths, weaknesses, and goals. Be active in the process, and ensure that the accommodations and goals outlined in the plan are specific, measurable, and attainable.

Remember, the IEP and 504 plan are designed to help your teen boy achieve academic success. By working collaboratively with your teen's educators and advocating for his needs, you can ensure that your teen boy receives the support necessary to succeed in school and beyond.

- **Working with Teachers and Other Professionals**

Working with teachers and other professionals can be crucial in helping your teen boy with ADHD succeed academically and socially. Here are some tips for how to work with these individuals:

1. **Establish open communication:** Establishing a good relationship with your teen's teachers and other professionals involved in his care is essential. Let them know you are committed to helping your

teen succeed and are open to feedback and suggestions.

2. **Share information:** Share information about your teen's ADHD diagnosis and other important information about his needs and challenges; this can help teachers and other professionals better understand how to support your teen.

3. **Collaborate on strategies:** Work with teachers and other professionals to develop strategies to help your teen succeed at school and home; this may include accommodations such as extra time for tests, preferential seating, or a homework tracker.

4. **Attend meetings:** Attend school meetings such as parent-teacher conferences, IEP meetings, and 504 plan meetings. These meetings are an opportunity to discuss your teen's progress, needs, and any changes that may need to be made to his support plan.

5. **Advocate for your teen:** Be an advocate for your teen and ensure his needs are

met. If you feel your teen is not receiving the support he needs, speak up and work with the school and other professionals to find a solution.

Remember, working with teachers and other professionals is a team effort. Collaborating and communicating openly can help your teen boy with ADHD succeed academically and socially.

Chapter 7
EMOTIONAL WELL-BEING

As parents of a teen boy with ADHD, it's crucial to prioritize his emotional well-being. ADHD can affect a teen's self-esteem, mood, and relationships, so this chapter addresses emotional well-being.

In this chapter, we'll discuss various strategies that can help your teen boy with ADHD develop emotional resilience, reduce stress and anxiety, and improve their overall well-being.

Whether it's coping with daily challenges, building social connections, or managing intense emotions, the insights in this chapter will help you guide your teen boy towards emotional stability and fulfillment.

- **Understanding Emotional Regulation in Teen Boys with ADHD**

Emotional regulation is the process by which an individual manages and responds to their emotions in an appropriate and healthy way. Emotional dysregulation is a common challenge for many individuals with ADHD, including teen boys. Teen boys with ADHD often struggle to regulate their emotions, leading to difficulties with anger management, mood swings, and impulsivity.

Understanding emotional regulation in teen boys with ADHD is critical for parents to provide support and guidance. One of the key features of ADHD is impulsivity, which can lead to impulsive behavior and emotional outbursts. Additionally, teen boys with ADHD often struggle with low frustration tolerance, leading to heightened emotional reactions to minor frustrations or disappointments.

You need to help your son develop effective coping strategies for managing his emotions; this includes teaching him how to identify his emotions, recognize triggers that cause emotional dysregulation, and develop healthy ways to manage them. You must also model effective emotional regulation strategies, such as deep breathing exercises, mindfulness practices, and positive self-talk.

Helping teen boys with ADHD regulate their emotions can also involve seeking professional help, such as therapy or counseling. These professionals can provide targeted strategies and techniques for managing emotions and provide a safe and supportive space for teens to discuss their emotions and experiences.

Overall, understanding emotional regulation in teen boys with ADHD is critical for you to provide adequate support and guidance. With the right strategies and resources, parents can help their teen boys with ADHD develop healthy emotional regulation skills and improve their overall well-being.

- **Strategies for Managing Emotional Outbursts**

Managing emotional outbursts can be challenging in parenting a teen boy with ADHD. However, there are strategies you will use to help your teen manage his emotions healthily.

One effective strategy is to help your teen recognize their emotional triggers, including situations, people, or activities that tend to cause emotional outbursts.

Once these triggers are identified, you can work with your teen to develop coping mechanisms and healthy responses to these triggers; this can include taking a break from the situation, doing deep breathing exercises, or finding a healthy way to express emotions through art or exercise.

Another strategy is to teach your teen skills for emotional regulation; this can include mindfulness practices, meditation, or cognitive-behavioral therapy. These techniques can help your teen learn to recognize their emotions and respond to them in a healthy way.

It is also important to model healthy emotional regulation as a parent; this can include using language to express emotions in a healthy way, taking breaks to calm down when feeling upset, and practicing self-care.

Finally, you should communicate with your teen's mental health professional or healthcare provider if their teen's emotional outbursts interfere with their daily life or relationships. They will be able to offer additional support or recommend medication to help manage emotional dysregulation.

Managing emotional outbursts can be a challenging but essential aspect of parenting a teen boy with ADHD. By helping your teen identify triggers, teaching them skills for emotional regulation, modeling healthy behavior, and seeking support when needed, you will help him learn to manage his emotions healthily.

- **Helping Your Teen Boy Build Self-Esteem and Confidence**

As a parent of a teen boy with ADHD, it can be challenging to see your child struggle with low self-esteem and confidence. ADHD can make it difficult for your teen boy to excel in certain areas of his life, leading to feelings of inadequacy and frustration. However, it is possible to help your teen boy build self-esteem and confidence, which can lead to a happier and more fulfilling life.

One of the most important things you can do to help your teen boy build self-esteem and confidence is to influence his life positively. Encourage your teen boy to pursue his passions and interests, and support his efforts. Praise him for his achievements, no matter how small, and offer constructive criticism when necessary. Show your teen boy that you believe in him and his abilities.

It is also important to help your teen boy develop a positive self-image. Encourage him to focus on his strengths rather than weaknesses and help him see himself as a capable and worthy individual. Avoid comparing your teen boy to others; instead, focus on his strengths and abilities.

Another way to help your teen boy build self-esteem and confidence is to provide him with opportunities to succeed. Encourage him to try new things, take risks, and help him to set achievable goals. Celebrate his successes when he achieves these goals and encourages him to set new ones.

In addition, it is essential to help your teen boy develop effective coping mechanisms for dealing with stress and frustration. Teach him how to manage his emotions and encourage him to seek help. Please help him to develop healthy habits such as exercise, mindfulness, and adequate sleep, which can all contribute to better emotional well-being.

Finally, it is essential to remember that building self-esteem and confidence is a process, and it may take time for your teen boy to see improvements. Be patient and continue to provide him with support and encouragement along the way. With your help, your teen boy can develop the self-esteem and confidence he needs to thrive.

- **Coping with Anxiety and Depression**

Adolescence is a time of significant physical and mental change, which can be particularly challenging for teenagers with ADHD. Many teens with ADHD struggle with emotional regulation, which can lead to feelings of anxiety and depression. It is essential for you to recognize the symptoms of anxiety and depression in your teen boy with ADHD and to seek help as needed.

Some common anxiety symptoms in teens with ADHD include constant worry, difficulty sleeping, irritability, and physical symptoms like

stomach aches and headaches. Symptoms of depression may include:
- A persistent feeling of sadness.
- A lack of interest in activities.
- Changes in appetite or sleep patterns.
- Thoughts of self-harm or suicide.

There are many strategies that you can use to help your son cope with anxiety and depression. One crucial step is to create a supportive and accepting home environment where your son feels comfortable talking about his feelings.

Encourage your teen to express his emotions through healthy outlets, such as talking to a trusted friend or adult, writing in a journal, or engaging in physical exercise.

It is also helpful to teach your teen relaxation techniques, such as deep breathing, meditation, or yoga, which helps to reduce feelings of anxiety and stress. Suppose your teen is struggling with severe anxiety or depression. In that case, seeking professional help from a mental health provider may be necessary.

Remember that coping with anxiety and depression is an ongoing process, and there may be setbacks along the way. However, by providing a supportive and understanding environment and teaching your teen coping skills, you can help them develop the resilience they need to manage their emotional well-being.

- **Supporting Positive Relationships with Family and Peers**

Supporting positive relationships with family and peers is crucial for the emotional well-being of any teen, particularly for those with ADHD. Teens with ADHD often struggle with social skills, making developing and maintaining positive relationships challenging. Here are some ways to support your teen boy in building healthy relationships:

1. **Encourage social activities:** Encourage your teen to participate in social activities such as sports, clubs, or community

service. These activities provide opportunities to meet new people and build positive relationships.
2. **Model healthy communication:** By actively listening to your teen, healthily expressing your emotions, and practicing conflict resolution skills.
3. **Teach social skills:** Teach your teen social skills such as making eye contact, active listening, and appropriate body language. Practice these skills with your teen in role-playing scenarios.
4. **Encourage positive self-talk:** Encourage your teen to use positive self-talk and focus on their strengths; this can help build confidence and self-esteem, essential for healthy relationships.
5. **Set boundaries:** Encourage your teen to set boundaries in their relationships and teach them to say "no" when necessary; this can help them avoid unhealthy relationships and build positive ones.
6. **Seek professional help:** If your teen struggles with social relationships,

consider seeking professional help from a therapist or counselor. They can work with your teen to develop social skills and support building healthy relationships.

Remember that building positive relationships takes time and effort. Encourage your teen to be patient and persistent, and offer support and guidance.

- **Navigating the Challenges of Puberty**

Navigating the challenges of puberty can be difficult for any teen boy, but those with ADHD may face additional hurdles. Puberty brings many physical, emotional, and social changes that can overwhelm any adolescent. Still, these changes can be particularly challenging for those with ADHD.

During puberty, hormones surge, leading to mood swings, impulsivity, and increased risk-taking behaviors. Teen boys with ADHD may experience even more significant mood swings, anxiety, and impulsivity due to the disorder's nature. It's essential for parents to recognize that these behaviors are not intentional but a result of hormonal and neurological changes.

Additionally, social skills become more critical during puberty as teens navigate more complex relationships and social situations. Teen boys with ADHD may struggle with social cues, have difficulty reading social situations, and may act impulsively in social situations, leading to misunderstandings and social isolation.

You will be helping your son navigate the challenges of puberty by providing him with support and guidance. It's essential to educate him about the changes he will experience during this time and provide him with coping mechanisms to manage his emotions and impulsivity.

Encouraging positive relationships with family and peers, providing a structured routine, and helping them build self-esteem can also be helpful.

If your teen boy with ADHD struggles during puberty, seeking help from a mental health professional is essential. A therapist can provide additional support and guidance to help your teen manage their emotions and navigate the challenges of this developmental stage.

Chapter 8
PLANNING FOR THE FUTURE

The teenage years can be challenging, especially for those with ADHD. As a parent, you want to help your teen boy with ADHD navigate this time in his life and set him up for success; this includes helping him plan for the Future and prepare for the challenges ahead.

This chapter will explore strategies for planning for the Future, including setting goals, identifying strengths and weaknesses, and preparing for adulthood. By taking an active role in your teen boy's future planning, you can help him build the skills he needs to succeed in school, work, and life.

- **Preparing for Life After High School**

Preparing for life after high school can be challenging for any teenager and incredibly challenging for those with ADHD. As a parent, it's essential to help your teen boy with ADHD plan for the Future and set realistic goals that align with his interests, abilities, and strengths.

Here are some strategies to help your teen boy with ADHD prepare for life after high school:

1. Encourage your teen to explore different career paths and interests. Help him research various careers and talk to professionals in those fields.
2. Work with your teen to set short- and long-term goals. Breaking down large goals into smaller, achievable steps can help your teen feel less overwhelmed and more motivated.
3. Teach your teen about time management and organization skills. These skills will be crucial for success in college, vocational school, or the workforce.
4. Consider seeking support from a career counselor, therapist, or other professionals who can help your teen explore his strengths and interests, set goals, and develop a plan for achieving them.

5. Help your teen learn about financial management and responsibility, including budgeting, saving, and managing credit responsibly.
6. Encourage your teen to build and maintain positive relationships with friends, family, and mentors. These relationships can provide emotional support and guidance as he navigates adulthood.
7. Help your teen explore post-secondary education options like college, vocational schools, or apprenticeships. Research these options together and help your teen choose the best path for his goals and interests.

By helping your teen with ADHD plan for the Future and set realistic goals, you can help him build the skills and confidence he needs to succeed after high school.

- **Post-Secondary Education and Training Options**

Preparing for post-secondary education or training is essential for teenagers with ADHD. Considering their unique challenges and strengths is essential when planning for their Future. There are several options available for students with ADHD after high school.

One option is college or university. While transitioning to college or university can be challenging for any student, it can be tough for those with ADHD. Therefore, it is important to start preparing for this transition early.

You should begin researching colleges and universities that offer support services for students with ADHD, such as tutoring, academic coaching, and counseling services. Additionally, you can reach out to disability services offices at potential colleges or universities to learn more about the available accommodations.

Another option is vocational or technical training. These programs offer hands-on training in a specific field, such as automotive technology or culinary arts. For students who struggle with traditional academic settings, vocational or technical training provides a more practical and engaging learning experience. Additionally, many vocational and technical programs offer smaller class sizes and more individualized attention.

Another option is gap year programs. These programs allow students to take a break from traditional academic settings and gain real-world experience through travel, volunteer work, or internships. Gap-year programs can particularly benefit students with ADHD who may benefit from a non-traditional learning environment.

You must begin exploring these options early on to ensure they have the necessary skills and support to succeed after high school. Students with ADHD may benefit from working with a guidance or vocational rehabilitation counselor to explore their options and create a plan for their Future.

- **Preparing for the Workforce**

Preparing for the workforce is an essential consideration for any teenager. Still, it can be incredibly challenging for those with ADHD. However, with the proper guidance and support, teens with ADHD can build successful careers that utilize their strengths and interests.

A critical step in preparing for the workforce is exploring potential career paths. Teens with ADHD may benefit from careers that allow them to work independently, utilize their creativity, or involve hands-on work. It's important to encourage your teen to pursue their interests and passions, as this can help them stay engaged and motivated in their work.

Another critical consideration is building essential job skills. Time management, organization, and attention to detail are all crucial skills for success in the workforce. You can help your teen develop these skills by encouraging them to take on responsibilities at home, such as managing their schedule or keeping their room organized.

It's also vital to consider accommodations that may be necessary in the workplace. Some teens with ADHD may benefit from accommodations such as flexible work hours, the ability to work from home, or access to noise-canceling headphones. Encourage your teen to speak with potential employers about any accommodations they need to perform their best.

Finally, providing emotional support and encouragement is crucial as your teen prepares for the workforce. The job search process can be challenging, and it's essential for your teen to feel supported and confident in their abilities. Please encourage them to seek out mentors or career coaches who can provide guidance and support along the way.

- **Building Life Skills for Independence**

As parents of a teen boy with ADHD, it can be challenging to prepare them for the Future and help them develop the necessary life skills to become independent. It's essential to start early and work on building these skills gradually, so they can be better equipped to handle the challenges of adult life.

One crucial life skill for independence is time management. Helping your teen boy with ADHD develop a schedule and a routine can be a significant first step. Please encourage them to use a planner or a smartphone app to keep track of appointments, deadlines, and tasks. It can also be helpful to break down large tasks into smaller, more manageable steps and assign specific deadlines for each step.

Another critical skill is financial management. Teach your teen boy about budgeting, saving, and making wise financial decisions. Please encourage them to get a part-time job or start a small business to gain valuable work experience and develop a strong work ethic.

Cooking and cleaning are also essential life skills for independence. Teach your teen boy how to cook simple meals and clean up after themselves; this will help them develop a sense of responsibility and self-sufficiency.

Social skills are also crucial for independence. Encourage your teen boy to participate in social activities and develop healthy peer relationships. Teach them how to communicate effectively and constructively resolve conflicts.

Finally, encourage your teen boy to set goals for themselves and work towards them. Whether learning a new skill, pursuing a hobby, or achieving a specific academic or career goal, having a sense of purpose can help them stay motivated and focused.

By working on these essential life skills, you can help your teen boy with ADHD develop the independence and self-confidence they need to succeed in adulthood.

- **Navigating the Transition to Adulthood**

Navigating the transition to adulthood can be a challenging time for any teenager. Still, it can be challenging for those with ADHD. As a parent, it's essential to help your teen boy with ADHD prepare for the transition and develop the skills and strategies necessary to become an independent adult.

One of the first steps in preparing for the transition is to start thinking about your teen boy's long-term goals and aspirations. What does he want to do after high school? Does he want to attend college or vocational school? Does he have a career in mind? By helping your teen boy identify his goals and interests, you can develop a plan for achieving those goals.

Another critical aspect of the transition to adulthood is developing life skills. These skills include time management, money management, and household management. It's essential to start teaching your teen boy these skills early on so that he can gradually develop independence and responsibility.

One helpful tool for teaching life skills is to use real-life scenarios and experiences. For example, encourage your teen boy to help with household chores like laundry or grocery shopping. You could also encourage him to get a part-time job or volunteer in the community. These experiences can provide valuable opportunities for your teen boy to learn new skills and build confidence.

As your teen boy prepares for adulthood, it's also essential to ensure that he receives any necessary support and accommodations; this might include continuing to work with teachers and other professionals to manage his ADHD symptoms or accessing support services through his college or vocational program.

Ultimately, the transition to adulthood is a complex process that requires careful planning and preparation. By working with your teen boy to identify his goals and interests, teach life skills, and provide ongoing support, you can help him navigate this challenging time and build a successful future.

CONCLUSION

As you reach the final pages of this book, it's crucial to recognize that parenting a teen boy with ADHD is a journey filled with both hurdles and triumphs. But amidst the **challenges**, there lies immense potential for **growth** and **transformation**.

You're not alone in this path. By taking proactive steps to understand and address your teen's ADHD, you're not just shaping his present, but also laying a strong foundation for his future success.

In the midst of chaos, remember to prioritize your own well-being. Only by nurturing yourself can you effectively nurture your son. By fostering open communication, empathy, and patience, you'll **forge** a bond that withstands any **obstacle**.

Your **teen** possesses a unique blend of talents and **capabilities** waiting to be unleashed. It's your role as a parent to guide him on this journey of self-discovery, encouraging him to embrace his strengths and overcome his challenges.

With each small victory, celebrate the progress made and **acknowledge** the effort put forth. And as you continue to support and uplift your teen, remember that your dedication does not go unnoticed. Your unwavering love and commitment are the driving forces behind his growth and resilience.

So, as you close this chapter, embrace the power of positivity and perseverance. Your journey with your ADHD teen son is just beginning, and with your steadfast guidance, he's destined to soar to new heights. Don't hesitate to share your experiences, leave a **review**, and inspire **others** on this transformative path. Empower your **teen** to **thrive** and embrace the endless possibilities that lie ahead with this book.

Other Books by the Same Author

1. **Raising Teenage Girls For Mom and Dad:** A Definitive Guide for Understanding Your Daughter's Development and Managing Your Teen Anger!

Dive into the complexities of parenting teenage girls with this comprehensive guide. From navigating their developmental milestones to managing teen anger, this book equips parents with the tools they need to support their daughters through the ups and downs of adolescence.

2. **Raising a Teen Boy with Oppositional Defiant Disorder:** An Empowered and Compassionate Handbook for Parenting Your ODD Teen

Parenting a teen with Oppositional Defiant Disorder (ODD) can be challenging, but this empowering handbook provides compassionate guidance. Learn effective strategies to support your teen and strengthen your parent-child relationship, fostering understanding and resilience.

3. **Empowering Your Teenager:** How to Understand, Support, and Inspire Your Teen Through Despair and Anxiety

In a world filled with despair and anxiety, empower your teenager to thrive with this insightful book. Discover practical tips and compassionate insights to help your teen navigate life's challenges with resilience and courage.

4. **Raising A Teen Girl With Anxiety:** Coping Skills For Raising Your Young Girl With Anxiety

Parenting a teenage girl with anxiety requires empathy and understanding. This book offers coping skills and strategies to support your daughter's emotional well-being, helping her build confidence and resilience in the face of anxiety.

5. Raising Teenage Boys For Mom and Dad: A Definitive Guide for Understanding Your Son's Development and Managing Your Teen Anger!

Understand your teenage son's development and manage his anger effectively with this definitive guide. Packed with practical advice and real-life examples, this book helps parents navigate the complexities of raising teenage boys with confidence and compassion.

6. Raising Teen Girls With ADHD: Overcoming the Challenges and Celebrating the Strengths of Your Daughter with ADHD

Celebrate the strengths of your daughter with ADHD while overcoming the challenges with this insightful book. Discover strategies to support and empower your teen girl, helping her thrive academically, socially, and emotionally.

Printed in Great Britain
by Amazon